THE ROOM
OUTSIDE

'Designing and creating a makeover garden with HammondCare for people living with dementia was challenging but extremely satisfying. That's why I am especially pleased to see this new book that's full of dementia design principles and practical advice. Access to gardens and outdoors is vital for all of us but especially for older people and people with dementia. We saw this ourselves in the garden we created and hope this book supports the development of many more dementia-inclusive gardens.'

Jason Hodges, Landscaper and designer, Better Homes and Gardens

'This straightforward and well-illustrated book distills the experience of many years of designing gardens for people with dementia. It provides an invaluable guide for anyone wanting to design an outside space which encourage people with dementia to go outside for a really positive experience.'

Professor Mary Marshall OBE

'It is widely accepted that gardens and gardening have a beneficial impact on our well-being, and our mental health in particular. People with dementia may need support through provision of the right environment and their needs should not be overlooked. As well as being a practical source of information, *The room outside* describes a range of case studies which demonstrate the value and the potential impact from being outdoors, simply being in gardens, or gardening. This is a clear and well-presented book that provides a plethora of ideas, examples and inspiration, with useful tips throughout.

Pam Whittle CBE,
former President of Royal Caledonian Horticultural Society

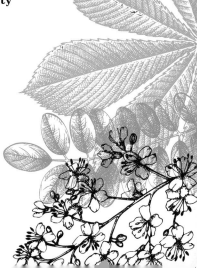

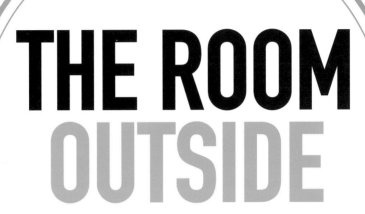

THE ROOM
OUTSIDE

Designing outdoor living for older
people and people with dementia

Annie Pollock *with* Colm Cunningham

DEMENTIA DESIGN ESSENTIALS

Published by HammondCare Media

Sydney, Australia, Edinburgh, Scotland.
hammondcaremedia@hammond.com.au
hammondcare.com.au
dementiacentre.com.au

ISBN 978-0-9945461-6-6

Design: Melissa Summers of SD Creative

 A catalogue record for this book is available from the National Library of Australia

Important: Dementia care knowledge and research is continually changing and as new understanding develops, so to does the support provided for people with dementia. All care has been taken by the authors and publishers, as far as possible at time of publication, to ensure information is accurate and up-to-date. The information in this book is not intended to be used to diagnose, treat, cure or prevent any disease, nor should it be used for therapeutic purposes or as a substitute for your own health professional's advice. The authors do not accept liability for any injury, loss or damage incurred by use of or reliance on the information contained in this book.

Thank you: HammondCare Media and the Dementia Centre are committed to providing excellence in dementia care. Older and younger Australians living with dementia deserve services that are designed and delivered based on evidence and practice-based knowledge of what works. This is achieved through providing research, training and education, publications and information, consultancy and conferences. Thank you to everyone who supported the publication of *The room outside: Designing outdoor living for older people and people with dementia*.

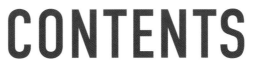

CONTENTS

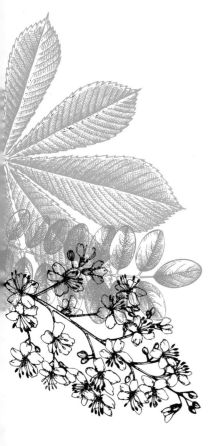

'...good design for older people and those with dementia also works for everyone, as many of us are impaired by the environments we live in.'

Opposite: Planters, Cyrenians Community Garden, Royal Edinburgh Hospital, Scotland.
Photo: Annie Pollock

INTRODUCTION

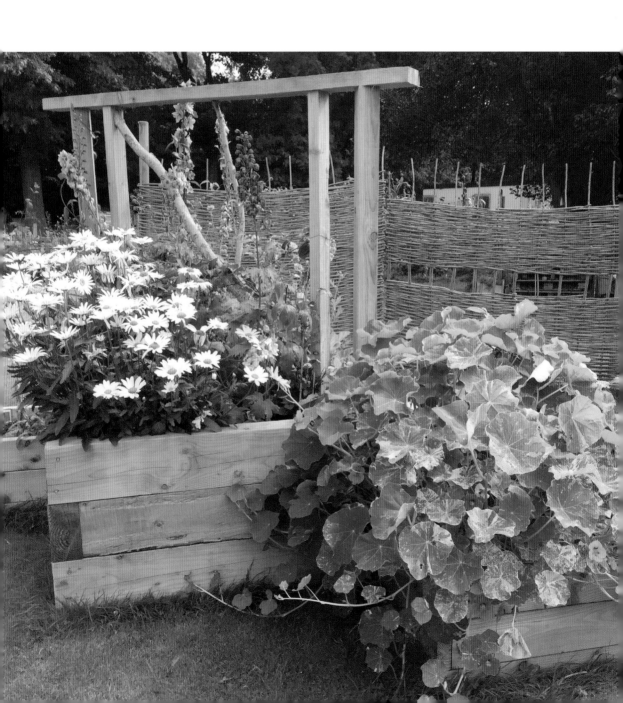

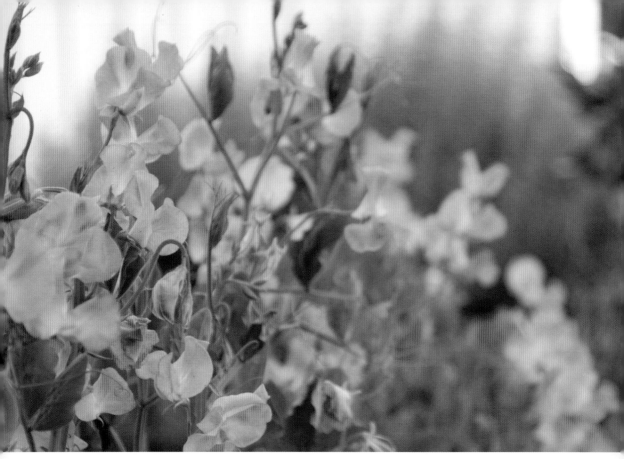

Sweet pea, probably the most popular annual flower, prized for colour and scent.

'Research and experience continues to show the significant benefits of an outdoor space to a person's physical and mental wellbeing.'

Extensive research shows the benefits of being outside for people of all ages and yet the need to provide a meaningful outdoor space for people with dementia is still not widely recognised. Many aged-care homes and hospitals do not support residents to have access to outdoors and even when they do, it may be a requirement to be accompanied! This access is often further limited by the outdoor spaces being inappropriate and/or unsafe for the needs of the people who live there.

Research and experience continues to show the significant benefits of an outdoor space to a person's physical and mental wellbeing. Not having this space limits and possibly denies the person positive, personalised and enriching aspects of care and will impact upon their general health. Significantly, for people with dementia, restricting outdoor access may lead to the person becoming confused, distressed and annoyed. This can have the negative result of the person being chemically (drugs) or physically restrained.

Recent groundbreaking research[1] in the UK has clearly shown that services providing care for older people should not only have appropriate outdoor spaces, but that these spaces should be readily accessible. This research highlights issues central to the purpose of our book:

> This large prospective cohort study provides new evidence to support the need for unrestricted access to outdoor space in care homes. The implications appear clear, access to outdoor space for residents too frail to access it, may worsen mood. If outdoor space is provided, care homes should ensure that care arrangements mean residents can actually access it.

Unlocked doors to outdoor space is not sufficient; care home design needs to enable residents to access outdoor space independently when possible and provide spaces that are safe, appropriate and comfortable for older people; and promote a culture that optimizes the use of outdoor space.

The room outside builds on international books on the topic (listed under 'References' and 'Further Reading') and expands on these to include:

- guidance on the design of outdoor spaces for older people with dementia that is relevant internationally

- details of the advantages of providing outdoor spaces in relation to health and wellbeing

- site layout to maximise the usefulness of outdoor spaces

- easy access and use of outdoor spaces for older people and those with dementia

- cultural and religious differences and how these might guide the design to be more appropriate for particular groups.

We hope that the outcomes of this book will be to:

- encourage the creation of outdoor spaces in care settings

- provide a better understanding about what makes outdoor spaces meaningful for people with dementia

- spur on those who have created suitable outdoor spaces for older people and people with dementia and encourage them to share positive outcomes.

Relevant for a variety of settings

While much of the book is focused on outdoor spaces for residential or hospital care, many of the principles will be applicable for respite and day settings and for people living at home with dementia and their family or carers.

For those who are working with existing care home or hospital buildings, even being able to provide just a small outside area that gets sunshine and fresh air is better than nothing. It can be easy to achieve a lot with little expense. For example, providing good outdoor seating, planters with colourful and seasonal planting, good signage (if required) that leads people to and around the outdoor spaces and perhaps some items of particular relevance to the residents, will all help to enrich your 'room outside'.

It's worth noting that good design for older people and those with dementia also works for everyone, as many of us are impaired by the environments we live in.

Being outside adds to everyone's quality of life, not least those with dementia. In the longer term, it may also reduce the need for drug treatment, create happier staff and reduce staff turnover, all of which can save money.

By writing a book that unites research into outdoor spaces for people with dementia, together with the 'nuts and bolts' of design it is hoped to enable people with dementia and older people rather than disable them which, sadly, is so often the case.

The authors hope the book will provide what is needed to create well-designed outdoor spaces, which enable people with dementia to access *The room outside* and to use, enjoy and be safe outdoors as part of an improved quality of life.

'Being outside adds to everyone's quality of life, not least those with dementia.'

Opposite: Enjoying the Better Homes and Gardens makeover at HammondCare Erina.

01
IMPAIRMENTS OF DEMENTIA AND OLDER AGE

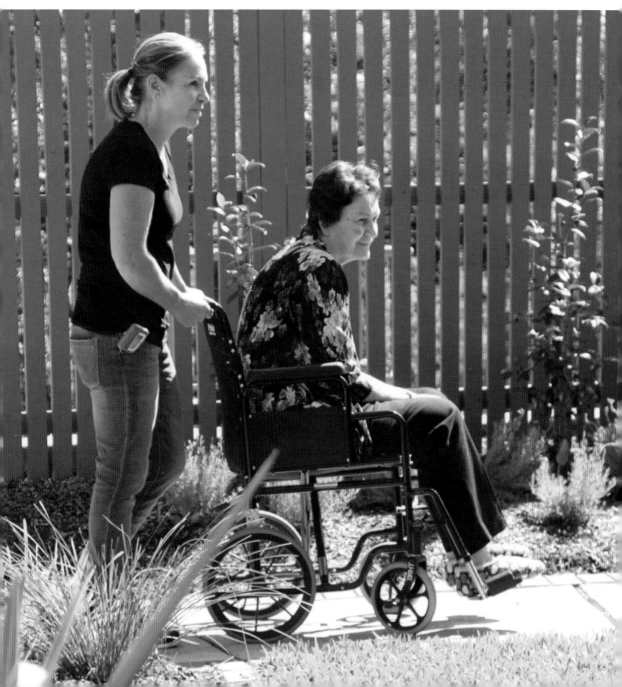

It is essential to understand that dementia is not only a condition impacting on memory, but affects the person's physical and psychological wellbeing. Progressive changes in a person's 'functioning' have traditionally been attributed to the inevitable decline of dementia. Increasingly it has been recognised that we need to investigate and treat other causes of change in the person's abilities. At times, dementia can simply make it harder for the person to identify what is causing the change, compensate for this or ask for help.

People with dementia will experience significant sensory challenges[2] and one example is hypersensitivity to sound. This can result in people with dementia being referred for 'behaviour management' for constantly walking away and leaving noisy and busy spaces.[3] When hypersensitivity is considered alongside the levels of noise in these spaces, then this 'behaviour' is not an unreasonable choice given the circumstances. Lack of access to the outdoors is routinely assessed as a contributing factor to the escalation of this 'behaviour' as an issue for the person and those supporting them.[4]

To help design enabling environments for people with dementia, it is vital to understand the impairments of dementia and the additional complexities when conditions of age are also present. We have to always think of the parallel sensory, physical and environmental circumstances impacting on the person.

Dementia

People living with dementia can experience a variety of impairments due to damage caused in the brain. These can include:

- impaired memory—both short-term and long-term memory
- difficulty learning new information
- poor concentration
- shorter attention span
- disorientation—time, dates, location
- difficulty identifying and naming objects
- word-finding difficulties
- difficulty planning and organising movements, including coordination
- difficulty with planning and sequencing steps to complete a task
- changes in personality and mood
- Visuoperceptual problems—not understanding patterns or tonal changes
- impaired judgement.

Older age

People living with dementia may also experience aged-related changes and impairments, which can include:

- hazy vision (e.g. a yellowing lens and impairments caused by glaucoma, cataracts and macular degeneration)

- poor hearing (e.g. presbycusis, an inability to hear particularly high pitch sounds)—hearing aids amplify all sound/noise, often causing further confusion

- diminishing efficiency of lung function, affecting breathing capacity

- diminishing muscle volume, affecting exercise tolerance

- impaired proprioception (perception of where one's body is and what it is doing)

- poor mobility and balance (e.g. shuffling gait, reduced sensation in feet, slower reaction to adjusting balance/centre of gravity)

- an increased need to go to the toilet because of less efficient pelvic floor muscles in women and enlarged prostates in men.

In addition to these, many people have illnesses, side effects of medication and other conditions.

Changes in experiences of smell, touch and taste are just some of the senses that can be altered. A pleasant perfume for one person could be perceived as foul odour to another, so we cannot assume the positive experience of fragrance in a sensory garden will be the same for each individual with dementia. Recent work by people with dementia has provided significant insight into changes in sensory perception.[5]

A complex design problem!

When the complex impairments of dementia are added to those of older age, the risk of a person becoming overwhelmed, frightened or increasingly dependent upon others is all too clear. This can be compounded by the possibility that a person with dementia may not recall that they have any of these issues and be unable to problem-solve how to overcome them or what to do about them.

If we do not provide an enabling and supportive environment for a person with dementia, they will experience a higher level of disability (referred to as excess disability), which in turn can negatively impact on their self-esteem, confidence and self-worth.

It is usually an unsuitable, confusing or debilitating environment that creates issues for a person with dementia— physically, cognitively and emotionally, rather than their dementia alone.

This is why creating enabling and supportive environments is one of the key non-pharmacological interventions.

'...creating enabling and supportive environments is one of the key non-pharmacological interventions.'

Because I can!

Being contained or restricted in where we can go can cause distress, frustration and even anger. This can be particularly acute for someone living with dementia, who may not understand the 'why' of these obstacles. The person can too often be labelled as challenging or of having 'behaviours or psychological symptoms of dementia' (BPSD).

Many of the reasons why one might want to go, and should go outside, are addressed in this book. For someone with dementia these reasons may include seeking to remove oneself from a busy noisy area, feeling confined, or seeking space to be free to walk and explore.

The starting point in having accessible outdoor spaces should be because the person with dementia has choice and freedom to move. Not providing this space and neglecting to make it intuitive for people with dementia to both locate and access, will cause frustration and possibly lead to behavioural distress and anger.

The Australian Government funds a national program, Dementia Support Australia (DSA).[6] This service provides advice and support when a person with dementia has a behaviour that is not understood. A significant proportion of referrals identify the need to access the outdoors as part of addressing the perceived behaviour. Currently there is nothing like this in the UK.

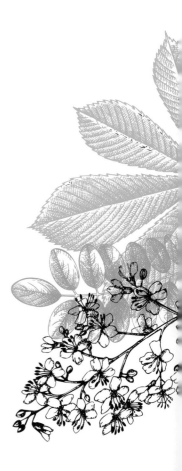

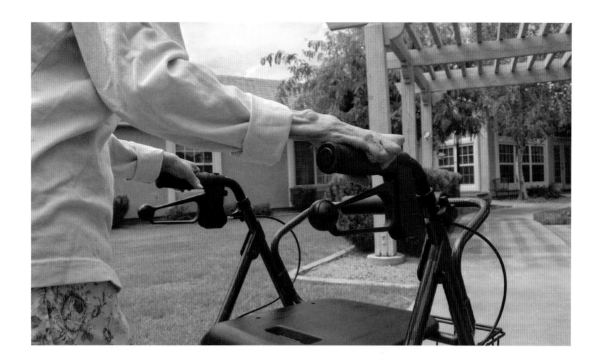

Case study 1
Unlocking the outdoor space

Nola had dementia and lived in a 15-bed aged-care home. A referral indicated that Nola's mood had changed since admission eight months previously. On referral to DSA, Nola was described as 'combative' and 'agitated' and examples were provided of her banging on doors and windows. The referral also stated there had been an incident several months earlier where Nola had successfully left the facility by standing on her four-wheeled walking frame and scaling a gate.

On assessment, it was identified that staff had been directed to lock the doors to the outdoor space, following Nola's 'absconding incident'. This was because staff reported they had a 'duty of care' to protect Nola from injury and potential harm. The decision impacted on everyone, as all residents were only allowed outside if a nurse was present. In reality, this meant that people got outside infrequently and only for short periods at a time. Nola's daughter and staff also reported that she now had increased night-time waking, walking and pacing around the care home, and agitation.

After a period of assessment, there was strong evidence that by locking the door to prevent a particular behaviour, this was adversely causing other behavioural symptoms for Nola. Moreover, the negative impact of not allowing access to the outdoor space is well supported in the literature with evidence-based design research finding that locked doors to outdoor spaces do increase distress and agitation. It was clear Nola's current lived experience was testament to this. Work was undertaken with the staff and family to reshape their thinking on assessing for risk and enabling choice and freedom of movement. The environment was also adapted, e.g. hiding and/or disguising the locked gate over which Nola had previously climbed. Emphasis was also placed on providing activities in which to engage Nola when outside, such as raised garden beds for her and others to enjoy. The doors to the outdoor space were unlocked again. Nola was no longer perceived as having 'behaviours', her mood changed and her sleep pattern improved.

Key points

- Dementia effects not only memory, but physical and psychological wellbeing.

- People with dementia will experience sensory challenges.

- Understanding the impairments caused by dementia and age-related changes is vital to achieving good design.

- Enabling environments which provide easy access to outdoors can reduce disability for a person with dementia.

- Restricting access and freedom of movement for people with dementia can be distressing and lead to being labelled 'challenging'.

- Accessible outdoor space which is intuitive to use promotes choice and freedom.

Opposite: Being outdoors is a healthy option. Nursing home at Chorley, Lancashire, England. Photo: Garuth Chalfont, Chalfont Design

02
GOING OUTSIDE IS
GOOD FOR US

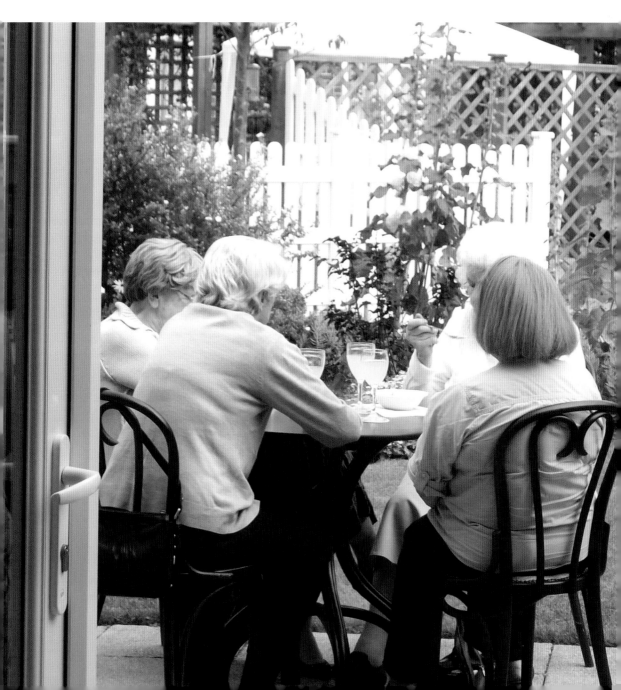

Being able to go outside is important for the mental and physical health of us all. For older people and people with dementia, in particular, easy access to suitable outside spaces is essential for many reasons including:

- improving general wellbeing

- helping stabilise circadian rhythms

- maintaining and improving fitness

- enhancing cognition through outdoor exercise

- encouraging socialisation and activity.[7,8]

Many older people and people with dementia can be overwhelmed by the noise and bustle indoors. The environment outside is often much more peaceful and being able to get outside can help people feel calm, reduce distress and associated behaviours.

Evidence obtained from people with dementia also suggests that they 'hope to maintain an ordinary way of life'[9]. Being able to go outside when one wants to, is an essential part of 'ordinary' life.

Conversely, not being able to go outside can be associated with depressive feelings[10], and indeed this may be partly due to being unable to escape from the noise and bustle inside the building.

There are many other reasons why being outside is so important for all of our physical and mental health and the following points provide an overview of the research in this field.

Exposure to sunlight

A recent study (Wright and Weller) provides a new perspective on the risks and benefits of sun exposure for older people, showing that 'inadequate sun exposure carries its own risks, and the older population are particularly sun deprived as recorded by low serum vitamin D levels and lack of outdoor activity'.[11]

While public health advice tends to concentrate on the dangers of sun exposure and the risk of skin cancers, 'advice on healthy sun exposure needs to be reconsidered, with reduction in all-cause mortality and morbidity as the primary end-point'.[12]

The same study notes that when Danish people who have had a non-melanoma skin cancer were compared with other Danes born in the same area and at the same time, it was found that the people with skin cancer were less likely to have had a heart attack, and less likely to have died of any cause. Similarly, a study of Swedish women showed that avoiding the sun was associated with a significant increase in deaths, with 3% of deaths connected to inadequate sun exposure. These findings, if applied to the whole Swedish population, would suggest that around 3% of all Swedish deaths are connected to inadequate sun exposure.

Effects of ultraviolet radiation

Ultraviolet (UV) radiation from sunlight varies in intensity and spectrum with season, latitude and time of day, and it has both beneficial and harmful effects on the health of older people.

The sunlight we receive consists predominantly of UV wavelengths categorised as UVA, UVB and UVC rays (UVC rays are prevented from penetrating our atmosphere by the ozone layer). UVA accounts for about 90% and UVB about 10%. Over-exposure to both types of rays is linked with skin cancers.[13] The important things to note in both include:

UVA rays

• are the dominant tanning rays

• are associated with skin ageing through over-exposure

• mobilise nitric oxide and can penetrate clouds and glass.

UVB rays

• vary in intensity according to season, location and time of day

• are the main cause of sunburn if a person's skin is over-exposed to direct sunshine

• trigger the production of vitamin D, but cannot penetrate glass.

There are ways to keep track of UV wavelengths. 'World UV', for example, is a smart phone app created by the British Association of Dermatologists in partnership with the Met Office, the national weather service for the UK. 'World UV', available for download from Goodle Play Store, provides a UV forecast for over 10,000 worldwide locations and the appropriate protection to take.

Importance of vitamin D

Vitamin D is essential for strong bones and muscle strength. In addition, there

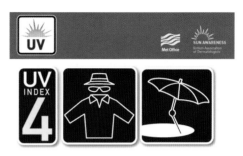

Your Risk Level

This exlpains what the risk is for the different skin types:

UV Index 3 and 4:

Medium risk for skin types 1 & 2.

Low risk for all other skin types.

Low risk for all other skin types.

Ways To Protect Your Skin Today:

Spend time in the shade between 11am and 3pm.

Protect your skin with clothing and a hat.

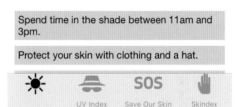

Screenshot of smart phone app 'World UV'.

is a growing body of evidence showing an association between low levels of vitamin D and illnesses such as multiple sclerosis, diabetes and cancer. 'Associated' in this context means that it is not known whether the lack of vitamin D is a contributing factor to the illness or if the illness itself leads to a lack.

Many people today are not getting enough vitamin D to stay healthy. Older people have thinner skin than younger people, which may mean they cannot produce as much vitamin D.[14] Other risk factors associated with lack of vitamin D are:

- living in the northern hemispheres, where there are fewer hours of over-head sunlight and the population generally lives further from the equator

- having darker skin

- obesity

- spending a lot of time indoors

- covering skin all the time (sunscreen and/or clothes).

Although there are natural sources in food (e.g. oily fish and eggs), the best and quickest way to get vitamin D is from the sun's direct rays during the summer months.[15] In northern latitudes, about 10-15 minutes in the sun with bare arms or legs can be enough for a very fair skinned person to make vitamin D, *before* putting on any sun protection—longer exposure is needed for people with darker skins. It is not necessary to tan and essential not to burn.[16]

In hotter countries such as Australia, a few minutes of sun exposure to the face, arms and hands should be sufficient, but it is important to avoid the middle of the day when the UV levels are at their highest. Further advice can be found on the Cancer Council Australia website.[17]

Even when the sky is overcast, the body can still make vitamin D, although a lot less.

Nitric oxide

Studies have shown that taking vitamin D supplements instead of having access to direct sunlight, does not demonstrate a reduction in malignancies. There is another component in the equation—nitric oxide.

Research carried out by the University of Southampton and The University of Edinburgh[18] found that exposure of bare skin[19] to sunlight mobilises nitric oxide from stores within the skin. This is significant because nitric oxide is crucial for maintaining healthy blood pressure, helps prevent atherosclerosis (arterial disease), and plays a role in modulating immune system function.

Mental illness, mood and cognition

There is increasing evidence that being outdoors in natural surroundings helps with improving mood. Wright and Weller (referring to a study by Kent et al[20]), note that 'Melatonin and serotonin regulation is influenced by sunlight and improvement in cognition is seen with increased sun exposure particularly in depressed individuals'.

A study by Mind.org[21] in 2007 showed the importance of sun exposure for mood when comparing exercise indoors and outdoors. Walking in indoor spaces such as shopping centres (or for the purposes of this book, perhaps care homes or hospitals) did not help improve mood or self-esteem. A 'green walk' on the other hand, reduced tension, frustration, depression and fatigue, with 88% of people feeling an 'overall improvement' from walking outside. In addition, a recent report by Natural England[22] looks at what people with dementia enjoy in the natural environment and the barriers that affect this. The most popular outdoor activity was walking.

A study in 2015[23] concluded that 'Allotment gardening can play a key role in promoting mental wellbeing and could be used as a preventive health measure'.

Evidence has also shown that depression caused by seasonal affective disorder (SAD) is greatly helped by exposure to bright light, although it does not necessarily have to be direct sunlight.[24] Another study suggests that bright light treatment and dawn simulation for those with SAD and bright light treatment for those with non-seasonal depression showed similar benefits to most antidepressant pharmacotherapy trials.[25]

Helping our circadian rhythm

Exposure to bright light helps our circadian rhythm to work properly and improves our sleeping patterns. It is not necessary to be outdoors for this to work, as natural light passing through glass is equally effective. Artificial lighting can also be useful, but it needs to be far brighter than would normally be found in a building—daylight is generally much brighter than artificial lighting.

A person's circadian rhythm is more liable to disruption with Alzheimer's disease. This may be partly due to insufficient sunlight, because exposure to morning daylight has been shown to help keep it working well. As Urrestarazu and Iriarte[26] note, 'During daytime, AD [Alzheimer's disease] patients should be encouraged to exercise regularly for at least 30 minutes and walk outdoors.'

Never too late to exercise

Another aspect of health and access to outdoors is the importance of exercise. Studies have suggested that regular exercise is associated with a delay in the onset of dementia and Alzheimer's disease, which supports the value of encouraging older people to exercise every day.[27] Of course, exercise also helps maintain general body health.

An article in the *New Scientist* in 2015[28] suggests:

> ...it's never too late to start. The hippocampus shrinks as we get older, leading to typical struggles with memory. But aerobic exercise not only prevents this loss—it reverses it, slowing the effects of getting older.

Breathing fresh air

Everyone needs oxygen—but for those people with impaired cognition, it is particularly important to get oxygen to the brain, and for those with impaired lung function, getting fresh air outdoors is also vital.[29] Outdoor air is normally much fresher than inside a building—carbon dioxide concentrations outdoors are generally around 400 parts per million whereas they can easily exceed 2000 parts indoors, affecting a person's cognitive function.[30] Where the outdoor air quality is poor, tree planting between a busy road and a care home can help improve quality (see Chapter 3).

Don't forget staff and carers

When discussing the health benefits of being outdoors, it's important not to forget those who work with and care for people with dementia. Being able to get some free time outdoors can dramatically increase positive mood, help prevent burnout from stressful working and reduce staff turnover. Staff and carers also need the health benefits of vitamin D and nitric oxide.

Outside access: the reality today

Despite all the known benefits of being able to get outside, a study carried out in Scotland in 2014 showed that in National Health Service units providing longer-term care for people with dementia, 'being outside is far from an everyday experience'.[31] The report noted that:

> ...only 71% of units had easily accessible gardens and only 37% of units had gardens which we considered to be safe, attractive and well maintained. We found that 53% of people had not been outside in the previous month even though it was summer.

Likewise in Australia, Theresa Scott's 2012 research[32] found that:

> Despite evidence for the healing benefits of contact with nature, for many older adults in aged-care facilities access to nature outdoors is very limited or non-existent.

A recent study by Stepchange[33] looking at care homes in England and Wales, found that the culture of the organisation was very important in determining the quality of the interactions with the outside:

> Those homes that had a fearful attitude towards Health and Safety tended not to be using their outdoor spaces to the optimal level for their residents. It was more difficult to spontaneously access the outdoors, staff lacked confidence in the outdoor environment and the homes were generally unprepared for interactions with the outdoor space. The care culture in operation influences engagement and activation levels too.

There are many reasons why staff may hesitate to access and facilitate the use of the outdoor space including:

- not understanding how important it is to be outside for good health
- being too busy—fearing that helping someone outdoors might be seen as skimping on their routine work
- not having enough staff to look after all those in their care
- feeling that the outdoor space is unsafe and being unable to oversee all the outdoor areas from within the building.

In the coming chapters, *The room outside* shows how to surmount most of these problems to ensure older people and people with dementia benefit from this wonderful, free, essential, pleasurable resource as much as everyone else. While we are looking mainly at design aspects of creating an enabling environment, it is vital that management is dedicated to a model of care that includes outside access and activities. Even the simplest garden area is beneficial if the staff encourage its use.

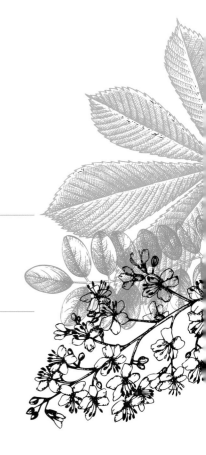

'Even the simplest garden area is beneficial
if the staff encourage its use.'

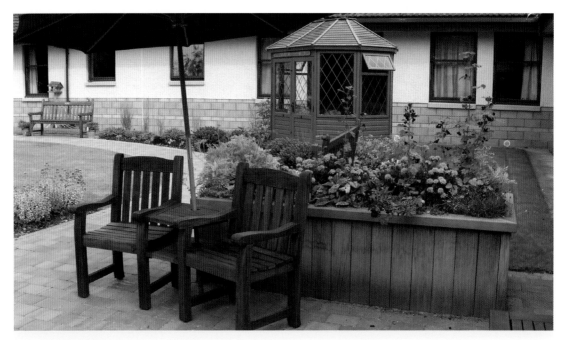

Garden at Crieff Community Hospital, Scotland. Photo: Annie Pollock

Case study 2
Crieff Community Hospital[34]

Michael* was admitted to Ward 1, due mainly to his carer's stress and a health decline in related to dementia. At home, he was a solitary man choosing to sit and watch TV with little or no interaction with anyone. Over time, his behaviour changed, causing his wife to be fearful and alarmed. Mainly due to Michael's history of alcohol abuse and physical and verbal aggression, he was initially admitted under the Mental Health Act as his family were extremely concerned that he would prove to be a 'handful' to manage.

As he was a heavy smoker, to avoid adding to his distress, we allowed Michael to smoke in the garden, either sitting on the garden benches or in the summerhouse. Very quickly this became his haven—he would head straight for the summerhouse in the morning with his papers and tobacco. He would welcome staff and others in to chat as if it was his own house.

He then started to take some ownership of the garden and was keen to sweep and do some other odd jobs. His family often commented that this was the best time they spent with him, being able to converse without constant arguments and repercussions.

Michael would spend hours chatting with staff about his youth. He also was very talented at playing the mouth organ and looked forward to being visited by the Elderflowers (a performing arts group dedicated to improving the

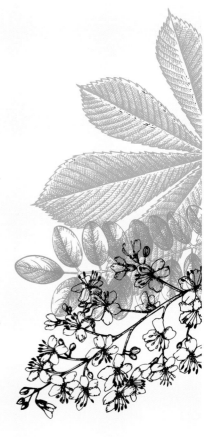

> 'My other vivid picture was Michael being very relaxed, watering the garden with an ice-lolly in his hand, chatting with staff and fellow patients.'

quality of life for people with dementia in hospital) and took great delight in trying to teach them how to play the mouth organ. On the days they came, the Elderflowers would approach the summerhouse, knock on the door and wait to be invited in—followed by lots of laughter. I could hear all this from my office!

My other vivid picture was Michael being very relaxed, watering the garden with an ice-lolly in his hand, chatting with staff and fellow patients.

It was vital to find the right care home for him on discharge—one that would allow him to access outdoor space as he had been doing and to ensure he wasn't cooped up indoors. Otherwise, there was a risk of further frustration and distress for Michael and his family.

The good news was that he was discharged to a local care home with a small secluded garden and a summerhouse, allowing care to continue with minimal disruption to his routine. The renewed connections with family members continued to grow and with transitional care carried out from the ward, Michael settled very quickly into his new home.

(*Name changed to protect privacy)
Diane Gardiner, SCN/Discharge hub co-ordinator.

Key points

- Access to outdoors helps people with dementia 'maintain an ordinary life'.

- Being outside allows production of vitamin D and nitric oxide and may elevate mood and strengthen circadian rhythms.

- Benefits of getting outdoors includes breathing fresh air and providing opportunities for exercise.

- Being outside in a 'green' environment elevates mood and increased sun exposure improves cognition, particularly in depressed individuals.

- All the benefits of the outdoor space apply to staff and carers, as well as the person with dementia.

- Other benefits include promoting calmness, confidence and multisensory stimulation.

- Apart from issues of design that arise from dementia and older age (covered in detail in chapter 6), the risk-averse attitudes of staff and management are very often the reason why outdoor areas are used so little.

Opposite: Even urban projects can feature outdoor spaces through careful planning, HammondCare, Wahroonga, Australia.

03
PLANNING FOR 'ROOMS OUTSIDE'

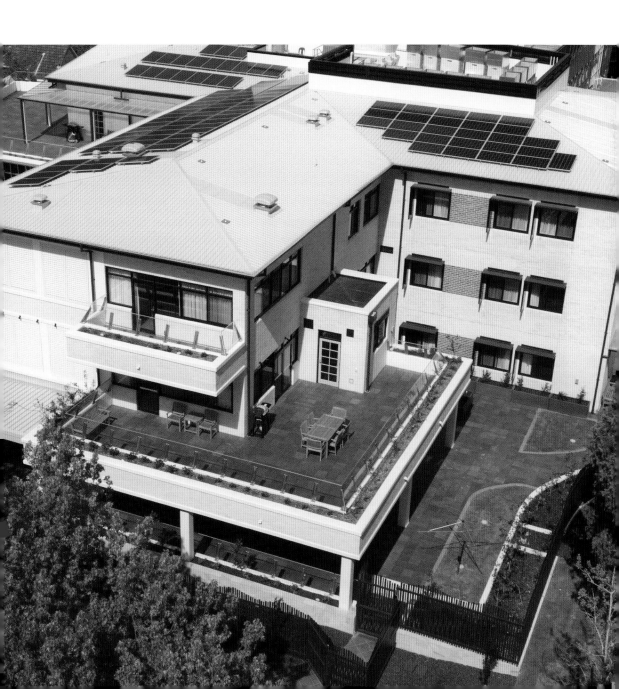

People adapt to the climates they live in. Their dwellings normally reflect their particular needs in ensuring a comfortable environment. However, with density, land cost and other commercial pressures, outdoor areas are increasingly ill-considered and treated more as 'left-over' space. If we want people to get outdoors, we must design outdoor environments that are comfortable and pleasant to be in— and ones that are also well-maintained.

At the very start of the project, it is vital to look at the site as a whole. As you do this, it is helpful to think of the outdoor space as a 'room outside', so that it's given the same importance as the rooms inside the building during early design stages. Leaving the outdoors as a 'left-over' space is often inadequate for people and plants alike.

As you develop designs for your building and its site, there is a range of important issues to consider.

Site context

It is always worth having a pre-application discussion with your local planning authority regarding the proposed building and its outdoor spaces. Make notes of the discussion points and circulate them among the design and management team. The following questions may need to be addressed when designing the outdoor areas:

• Is the site affected by any planning legislation? (In the UK and Australia it could be within a conservation area or next to a building of heritage value.)

• Are there trees within or just outside the site that are protected by the planning authority? Could any of these trees shade your proposed building, or perhaps even create a positive focal point?

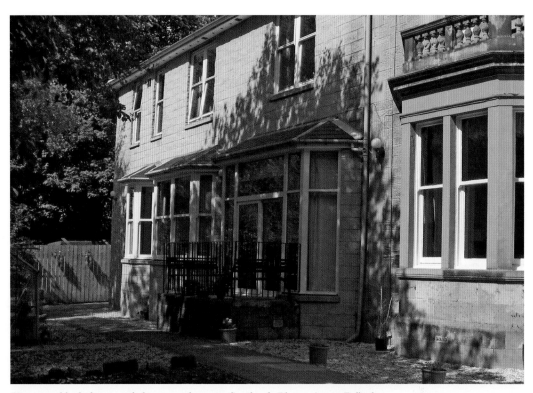

Trees can block direct sunlight: a care home in Scotland. Photo: Annie Pollock

- Consider whether the site is part of a 'Greenweb Restoration' (or similar) plan[35] which may impact the planting of non-indigenous plants in Australia. In the UK, if BREEAM (Building Research Establishment Environmental Assessment Method) accreditation on sustainability is required, this may also impact on planting design.

- Is there a busy road adjacent to the site that could lead to noise and air pollution?

- Are there sources of noise over which you do not have any control, e.g. aircraft? In this case, you might reconsider if the site is worth developing.

- Will there be a problem of 'overlooking' from outside the site— or from within the site to outside?

- If privacy or overlooking is not an issue, are there interesting things to look out on from within the building and the garden areas, e.g. a busy street or a school playground, which may help people with dementia retain contact with the outside world?

Consider orientation

Encourage the design team to produce sun access drawings so that you can see how much solar penetration there is to the outdoor areas at different times of the year.

Consider these options:

- Is it possible to create outdoor spaces on the sunny sides of the site? If so, use the sunless areas of the site for servicing and parking.

- If a sunny orientation is not possible, can the proposed building be low enough to allow sun penetration to the outdoor areas? Sun angles should be considered carefully along with the planned height of the building to ensure that direct sun can penetrate to ground level.

- Is there a site slope? This will affect sun access, the corresponding building height and width of outdoor spaces.

- Where do the prevailing winds come from? Consider providing outdoor shelters to provide a suitable microclimate for older people and people with dementia. Such outdoor spaces can often be used for outdoor events and an electrical supply can be useful.

Dealing with pollution

Many different types of pollution can affect the use of outdoor spaces. Noise and air pollution are two of the most obvious. Other types of pollution that may affect a site include:

- light, e.g. street lamps or shop windows

- visual, e.g. tall buildings, advertising hoardings, litter, site hoardings

- water, e.g. areas of stagnant water, poor site drainage, farm runoff.

Noise

Is there enough space on site to take the necessary action to mitigate outside noise, for example from a busy highway? Earth mounding or acoustic fencing may help with this.

The commonly held idea that trees and planting will reduce noise is rarely applicable, unless there is sufficient space available. Forest Research[36] notes that planting 'noise buffers' composed of trees and shrubs can reduce noise by five to ten decibels for every 30m width of woodland. To achieve this effect, the species and the planting design must be chosen carefully.

Air

A newly published study discovered toxic nanoparticles from air pollution in 'abundant' quantities in human brains.[37] This raises concern as recent research has suggested links between these magnetite particles and Alzheimer's disease, and air pollution has been shown to significantly increase the risk of the disease.[38]

If there is local air pollution, some trees can positively affect air quality, so tree planting may provide some mitigation if space on the site allows.

In the UK, a study by Lancs University[39] found that common alder (*Alnus glutinosa*), field maple (*Acer campestre*), larch (*Larix decidua*), Norway maple (*Acer platanoides*), scots pine (*Pinus sylvestris*) and silver birch (*Betula pendula*) were all shown to help.

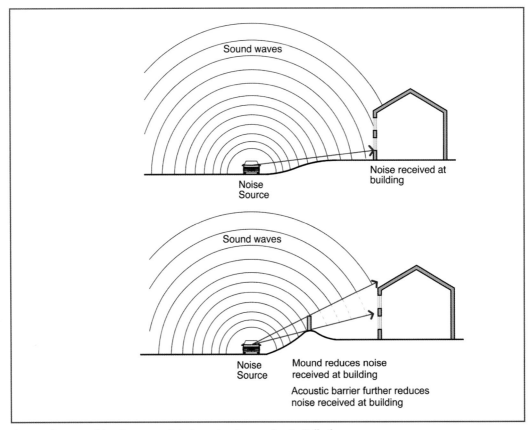

Appropriate sound barriers can minimise noise. Image: Annie Pollock

In Australia a recent study looked at air pollution in Sydney. The results showed that sites which had nearby green-space had lower particulates, even when pollutant sources were corrected for and factored into the analysis. Trees in the sample sites included Queensland brush box (*Lophostemon confertus*) London plane tree (*Platanus acerifolia*), black poplar (*Poplus nigra*), sweet gum (*Liquidambar styraciflua*) and green ebony tree (*Jacaranda mimosifolia*). There will also be different trees in other climatic area of Australia which help to reduce pollution, but so far the research appears to be limited.

Undoubtedly, there will be tree species in other countries that provide the same benefits. Being aware of the prevailing winds may help to determine the site layout and location of outdoor spaces.

Keep in mind also, that placement and selection of trees and plants is important, with a recent air pollution review by Abhijith[40] et al noting that:

> In a street canyon environment, high level vegetation canopies (trees) led to a deterioration in air quality, while low-level green infrastructure (hedges) improved air quality conditions. For open road conditions, wide, low porosity and tall vegetation leads to downwind pollutant reductions while gaps and high porosity vegetation could lead to no improvement or even deteriorated air quality.

'If we want people to get outdoors, we must design outdoor environments that are comfortable and pleasant to be in—and ones that are also well-maintained.'

Access to amenities and community

Being able to travel safely to local shops, cafés, libraries, post offices or places of worship can be so life enhancing for people in the earlier stages of dementia. Ideally the public environment and its amenities are dementia-inclusive. As towns and cities move towards adopting a dementia-inclusive status, we hope this will become normal design thinking. Having a local park nearby can also be a tremendous bonus, particularly if it's dementia-inclusive and has well signed public toilets.

Opportunities for community involvement

Contact with the surrounding community can be very rewarding. Not only does it keep the residents in touch with life beyond the care home, but facilities that can also be used by the community are usually more financially viable:

*   Is the site near a school? Visits from local school children can be welcome and outdoor spaces can provide many opportunities for activities, especially if they have verandahs, shelters, greenhouses or sheds.

*   Does the building itself have facilities that can be used by the community? Does it contain a café? A hairdresser/barber? Rooms for therapies or art classes? A room for concerts or cinema shows? All these facilities could be used by the wider community, offering further opportunities for social interaction between residents and the community.

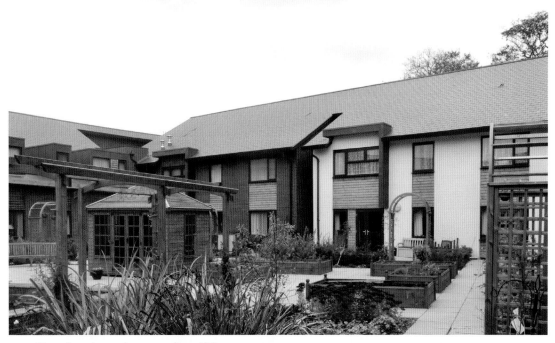

Shared gardens enhance quality of life.
Photos: Lisa Broom, Homes and Communities Agency, England

Case study 3
Oakland Swadlincote

In *The Derbyshire Telegraph* (March 20, 2013), a 99-year old woman
living at the care village, Oakland, in Swadlincote said:

> Everything is on the doorstep and you don't have to worry about things like
> cooking meals—the restaurant does beautiful food and the hairdressers is
> great... I'm very happy here—it really is out of this world.[41]

The article's further comments on the care
village included the following description:

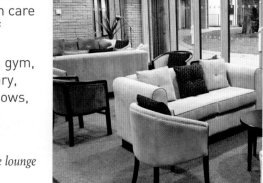

> With the elderly population soaring, the
> village was built to enable people with care
> needs to live independently with staff
> available on site all the time. It has a
> bar, restaurant, lounge area, IT suite, gym,
> jacuzzi, hairdresser, craft room, library,
> landscaped gardens and a hall for shows,
> dancing, bingo and films.

View from the lounge

Key points

- Make a careful analysis of all site issues at a very early stage, including surrounding amenities.

- Ensure that this analysis informs the design so that outside areas are not just 'left over' space but 'rooms outside'.

- Consider outside space as a 'room outside', linking with internal rooms in a sensible way.

- Maximise daylight and sunlight access.

- Allow for sheltered outdoor areas, e.g. sheds, gazebos, verandahs and covered walkways.

- In addition to the residents, consider how the wider community might contribute and benefit from outdoor spaces.

- Consider air quality and how this might be improved if necessary.

Opposite: Shed and potting area, St Catherine's View, Colten Care, Winchester, England.
Photo: Annie Pollock

04
DEVELOPING A RANGE OF ACTIVITIES

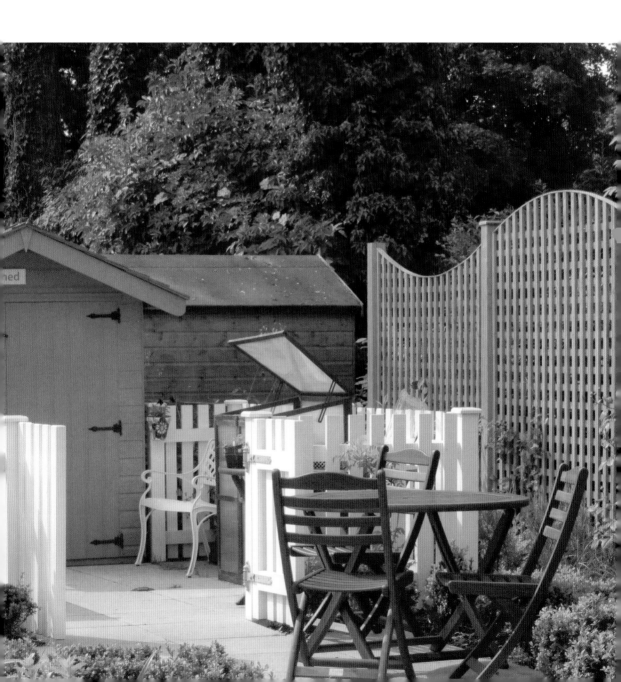

A study by Natural England in 2016[42], reported that 'engaging in outdoor activities that have a purpose and those that involve being with other people provide the greatest motivation for people living with dementia'. The following were very popular—informal walking outdoors (38%) and wildlife or bird watching (25%).

This report noted the main barriers that inhibit older people from engaging in activities. Although these are in relation to being out in the wider community, they are relevant here too. These barriers are:

• lack of confidence

• fears and safety concerns

• insufficient information about what places have to offer and their suitability for visitors with dementia

• lack of support to get to locations

• lack of support to use facilities and to participate in outdoor activities

It's important to be aware of these barriers when designing spaces and activities to suit a diverse range of people, so please keep them in mind as you read through this book.

Types of outside space

Outside spaces for people with dementia need to be familiar and meaningful, which will help users feel more confident. The design must provide for a range of activities, which staff can help and encourage those they care for to be involved in. Outdoor areas are not 'show gardens' just to be looked at and admired.

Terms used to describe outdoor spaces, such as 'healing', 'sensory' and 'therapeutic' should be viewed as components of any outdoor space for people with dementia, although they have been used on occasion to describe a single garden.

'Healing' and 'sensory' are often used to describe gardens for people who are or have been ill, have dementia or other cognitive impairments. As people with dementia are likely to have failing senses (sight, hearing, memory), designs that can stimulate and appeal to the senses are clearly beneficial.

'Therapeutic' usually means providing appropriate things to do that in turn may improve mental and physical health. This might include supervised outdoor physiotherapy, which can easily be provided by simple garden tasks that are supervised by a trained therapist.

Garuth Chalfont (in his *Dementia Greencare Handbook*[43]) uses the following classifications for different types of outdoor spaces according to use:

• passive: a space that encourages calm, peace and rest

• active: a space designed to stimulate and enable active engagement

• risk-free: a space which people with dementia can use independently, but it is clearly visible from inside the building

- risk-assumed: a garden only used when accompanied by a member of staff, friend or other responsible person.

This is a sensible way of grading outdoor spaces, which in turn relates to the type of activity. We would add another variation—depending on the stage of a person's dementia, some people may be very able to safely use areas that are not observed or supervised. Indeed this may be particularly beneficial for a person's wellbeing as a place for relieving frustrations or escaping from noise and bustle.

We all need time out—and day care centres, care homes and hospitals are all particularly busy and noisy. Outdoor spaces can provide a haven of peace and quiet for escaping from this cacophony, in most cases (but not always), balanced against the need for supervision and visibility. Peaceful areas are also useful for sitting with friends, having a cup of tea or coffee, watching or engaging in an activity, doing a crossword, reading a book—all the normal things of everyday life.

We also need places in which to be active. For people with dementia, everyday activities that they have done in their younger lives are helpful—hence the need to research the background of the people for which you are designing.

To achieve these aims, considerations that are important include:

- wayfinding—paths need to be easy to follow and lead you back to a recognisable part of the building

- pleasing things to look at, touch and smell along the route

- things to listen to, such as the rustle of leaves and birds singing

- triggers for memories—items of particular relevance to residents or patients, such as an old car or tractor, a piece of workplace equipment, a fountain, artwork, particular plants, animals and items that might stimulate memories of picnics and barbecues.

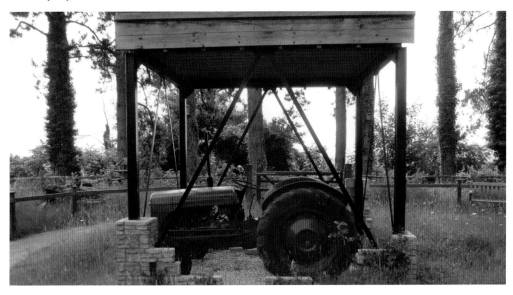

Memory trigger, St Catherine's View, Colten Care, Winchester, England. Photo: Annie Pollock

Activities to consider

Activity-based clubs can be a great way of involving people with dementia, but it is very important to know the background of your users and their interests. People may have a variety of pastimes, sometimes related to what they used to do during their working life and sometimes new ones embraced in retirement. Most people with dementia don't want to sit around being waited on and having nothing to do—boredom is a killer! Familiarity is key—spaces and actvities people can relate to.

The list of possible activities is almost endless and should be discussed at the briefing stage, however they might include any of the following:

Passive activities

- doing a crossword, reading a book, painting a picture—for which the bright outdoor light is helpful

- quietly chatting over a cup of tea or coffee, with plenty of chairs, tables and parasols if required

- table-based activities such as touching and enjoying plants and herbs—making herbal remedies such as 'bath treats'

- reflection, spiritual sustenance, praying.

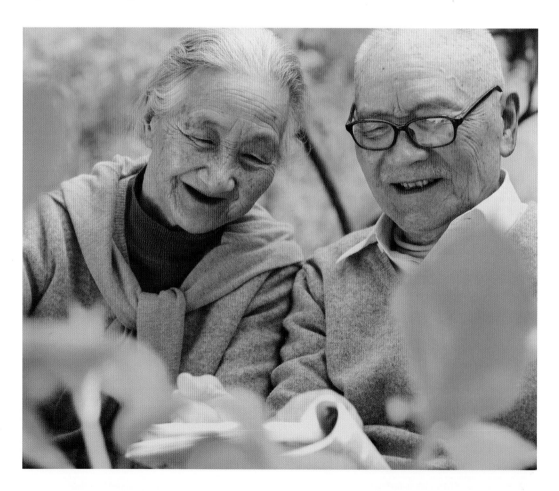

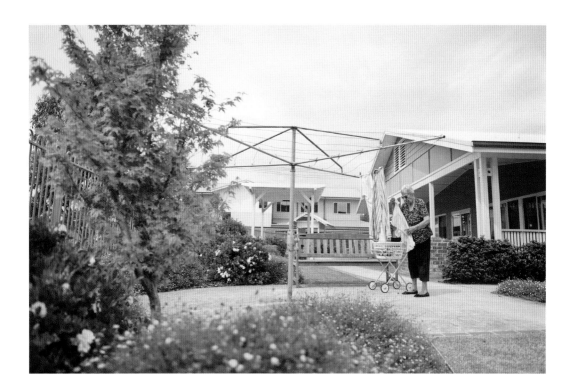

Energetic activities which may require staff involvement

- light gardening, for which raised planters and greenhouses offer many opportunities

- looking after small animals e.g. chickens, rabbits, birds for which hutches and enclosed runs are needed

- walking to destination points or an activity centre

- looking at and recording nature

- games, such as bowls, petanque, croquet, putting

- mending and making things, for which a garden shed is useful

- cleaning a car or motor bike (made safe, of course, with no engine!)

- hanging up clothes to dry or air, clothes poles or a rotary dryer, whichever is the most familiar

- helping set-up picnics and barbecues, which can also help stimulate appetite.

Caring for animals

Caring for animals will be familiar to many older people and a good example is the keeping of chickens. You may even have a friend who, when they visit, brings some of their home laid eggs. While it is important to consider guidance and regulations that may inform the keeping of chickens in an aged-care home, beware of the common myth that you cannot have chickens in residential care. Get to know the regulations well, as there are many examples of aged-care homes that keep chickens (and indeed other animals) with the involvement of residents!

One example of overcoming this perceived regulation barrier came about when an aged care home with chickens began to use the eggs in the food prepared for residents. Upon investigation, a number of criteria need to be met for these eggs to be used. The regulations required the following:

- the home had to be registered to produce eggs

- there had to be an annual inspection for the chickens' welfare, and

- eggs had to be date stamped for shelf life.

What appeared to be a barrier was easily overcome and once the care home had complied with the regulations for the keeping of chickens and the production of fresh eggs, they had created a meaningful activity for residents that contributed to the life of the facility both outdoors and in!

Accessible gardening

At this point, it is worth mentioning the 'The Creating Conversations Kit: Gardening'[44], developed over two years, and tested and evaluated by researchers at the Gerontology Department at Stirling University, Scotland. This can be easily delivered by care staff and activities organisers. It's a table-based activity which encourages meaningful engagement and getting to know the person with dementia—with the aim of stimulating memories of gardens and garden activities. This can then lead to activities outdoors, based on the conversations.

Health-related activities

- Light physiotherapy, which might require an area with a gentle incline and handrails for specific exercise.

- Space for group activities such as Tai Chi.

Activities for young visitors too

Play equipment for visiting children, or other all-age fun activities, can provide interest and participation. Clearly though, these must be safe for people with dementia too.

Building in adaptability

It's important to note that outdoor spaces need to be adaptable and this should be part of the brief. This is because:

- plants are living things that change with time

- residents and staff come and go

- different generations will have different memories and different associations with outdoor space

- the cultural mix of residents might also change with time.

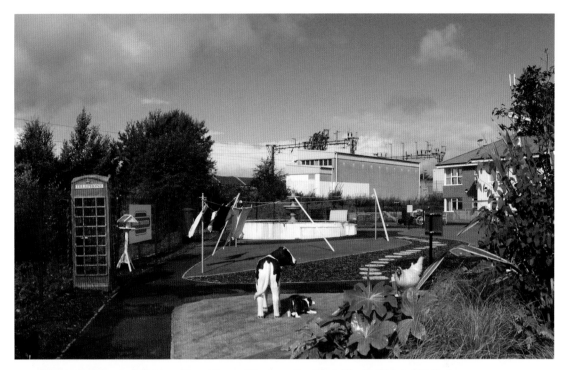

View of garden at 3 Bridges Care Home, Glasgow, Scotland. Photo: Richard Pollock

Case study 4
3 Bridges Care Home (Northcare), Glasgow[45]

3 Bridges Care Home has a grassy park-like section with a fountain and benches, a green area for bowls and skittles, a farmyard section with animals and an area for growing vegetables.

Young visitors to the home (i.e. grandchildren) have enjoyed the use of the children's play area when the weather permits, so instead of the children not looking forward to coming to visit a care home, most look forward to going along with their grandparents to the play area with swings, a chute [slide] and even a Wendy house [playhouse]. This area has given our clients a venue to spend time with their grandchildren where they can play. We have plenty of seating so they can see and enjoy and be part of their grandchildren's lives. This has enhanced the residents and the children's lives through play.

Jeff* who had not been out of his home for nine months before coming to the care home due to his condition, had previously loved to play bowls. Now, he enjoys the activity garden, and is out in the garden playing bowls at every opportunity (only the rain stops play) with his family and friends. This has given him a new lease of life and he has made friends through bowling as other clients joining in.

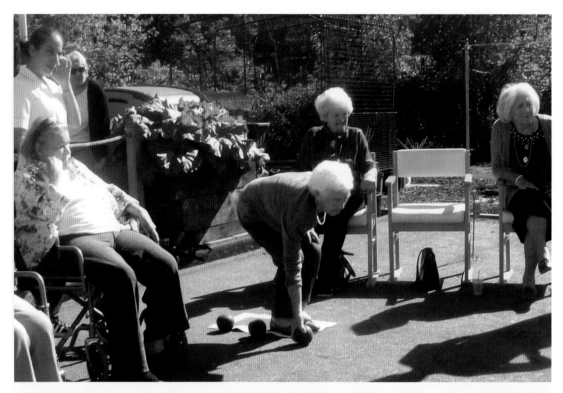

Playing bowls on a sunny afternoon. Photo: Northcare (Scotland) Ltd

'If the weather is inclement, she watches the chickens being fed by our pet carer, as she eats her breakfast. Our chickens and pigs roam free in the garden at this time in the morning.'

Jenny* who lives with dementia was very depressed before coming into 3 Bridges—now she is keen to be up in the morning to assist us with feeding the chickens. If the weather is inclement, she watches the chickens being fed by our pet carer, as she eats her breakfast. Our chickens and pigs roam free in the garden at this time in the morning.

George* loves to go in the garden and walk around the areas. He also enjoys being outside when the pigs and chickens are out. He is much more animated around the animals and this is echoed when he returns into the home.

Ethan* who lives with dementia, used to be a postman, enjoys going out to check the post box in the garden. This gives him a sense of purpose as he was a great postie.

(*Name changed to protect privacy)

Case study 5
Willow Cottage, The Meadows, (HammondCare), Hammondville NSW, Australia[46]

We often bring our grandchildren to visit their great grandmother and find that many of the same features that make the cottage outdoor spaces interesting but safe for the older generation do the same for all of us. The subtly enclosed outdoor area backs onto a pond where we can safely feed the ducks (and eels and turtles!) from a familiar, fenced platform with no steps involved. The children might also ride scooters along the level, well-defined paths while we sit and enjoy a picnic. Watering newly planted flowers, picking lavender and sharing the fragrance are among favourite pastimes for the young and the young at heart.

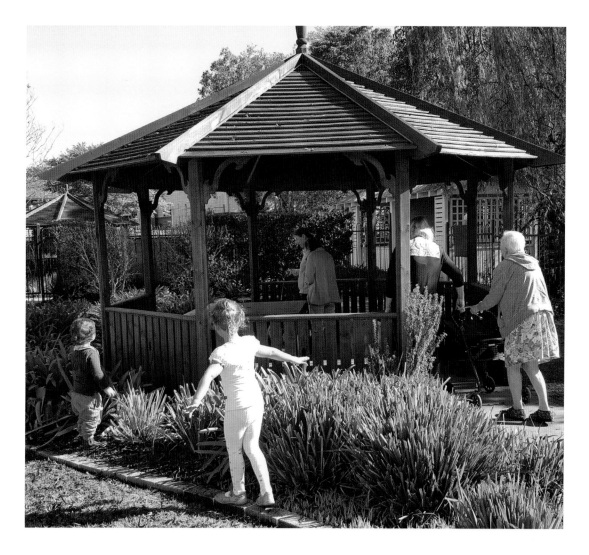

Key points

- Create outdoor spaces that are familiar and meaningful to the users —don't design a 'show garden'.

- Think about how the garden will be used and the attributes to include in the design.

- Provide activities that are relevant to the people with dementia and their background.

- Ensure a degree of adaptability.

Opposite: A helping hand to get outside, HammondCare, Erina.

05

DESIGN THAT HELPS PEOPLE GET OUTSIDE

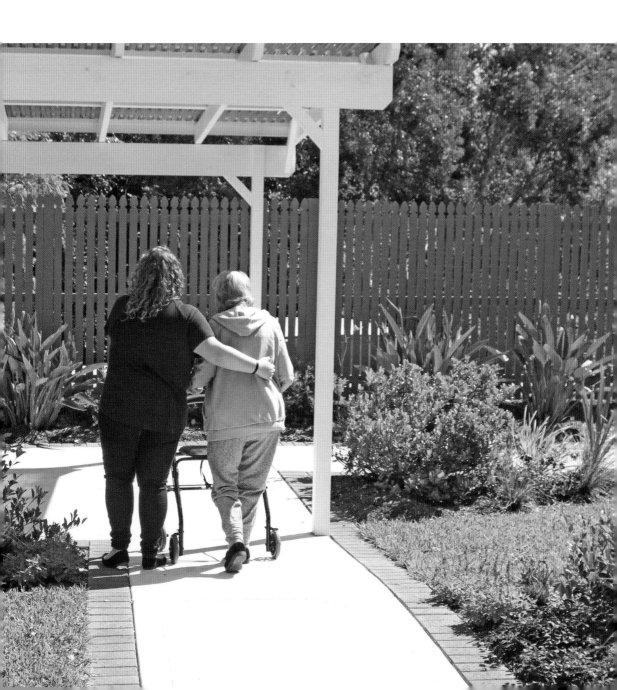

There may be many reasons why people with dementia don't go outdoors. Those related to age, dementia or staff attitudes have been covered earlier. This chapter looks at the simple, positive design measures that can help reduce obstacles to getting outdoors, many of which are created by the design of the environment.

Solving common design obstacles

It is easy to take for granted things we use every day such as entries and doorways. A closer look at these everyday functions may reveal subtle barriers for people with dementia:

- Even if the door to outside is un-locked, it may still have a security alarm, which can cause distress to residents if it activates—so it is vital that alarms are used only when an action may cause someone to be unsafe (or better still, silent pagers alerting staff when someone is at risk).

- The nearest way out may be a fire door and staff discourage people from using it—so ideally fire doors should be disguised or not easily seen by people with dementia. Signage that is intended to help staff operate fire doors could (with fire safety authority permission) be located higher up on the door, out of easy view for older people (such as 'push bar to open door').

- People with dementia may not be able to locate the door because its design is too similar to the adjacent windows. So ensure that doors leading to garden areas are easy to see, find and operate and contrast tonally with any adjoining windows or walls by no less than 30 light reflectance value (LRV). See more detail on this issue on page 52 'Surfaces that are enabling'.

- The door handle is hard to use and/or difficult to see—so use a comfortable 'U-shaped' lever handle in a contrasting tone to the door.

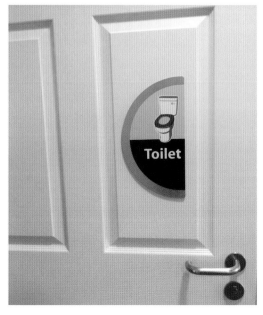

An easy-to-use U-handle door lever.
Photo: Richard Pollock

- Accessing the outside areas is diffi-cult—there may be steps, high thresh-olds, and/or strong tonal contrasts between inside and outdoor surfaces. Ensure there is a ramp if required and no floor/paving contrasts greater than 5 LRV.

- There is no visible or nearby toi-let either outside or just inside the building—could an outdoor toilet be constructed? If not, good clear signage to the nearest existing toilet may help solve the problem.

- The views outside are obscured by planting—remedy this by cutting back vegetation or replanting.

- The views outside are obscured by the window design—can the design be amended or the windows replaced?

- People living on the first floor and above may have no outdoor space and cannot manage the stairs or lift to ground level—could a balcony be constructed? Is there an area of flat roof that could be strengthened and converted to a roof terrace? Could the lift down to ground floor be made dementia-inclusive with clear controls, no mirror and a floor tone that matches the floor outside the lift?

There are nearly always design solutions to such problems. However, sometimes an existing building may pose some insoluble issues and you have to ask yourself if it is time to consider a more radical solution, such as major works.

Where a freely accessible and safe outdoor space is provided, the most common reasons given for not going outdoors are weather-related[47]:

- too cold or too hot
- too windy
- it has rained, is raining or is going to rain.

These conditions affect us all, but older people generally, including those with dementia, are often more sensitive to heat, cold, rain and wind. Providing effective outdoor shade and shelter, covered walkways and a comfortable place for putting on and taking off outdoor clothing will encourage many people to venture out, even in less clement weather.

There is no reason why people with dementia should be any more likely to come to harm outdoors than inside the building—it is all about getting the design right. The detail of this is discussed in the next chapter.

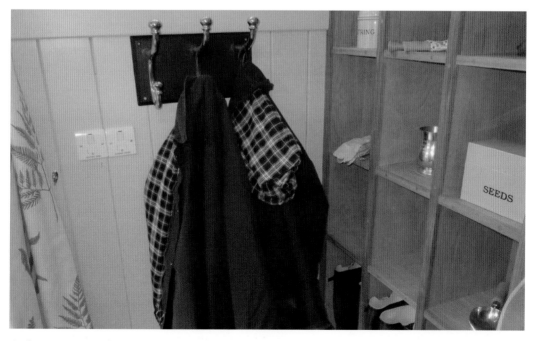

A place to store outdoor clothes, St Catherine's View Care Home, Colten Care, Winchester, England.
Photo: Annie Pollock

Where to locate outside access

A key to helping people get outdoors is the location of access. Deciding which rooms need direct access to outdoors may depend on the size, range of functions and usage of the building.

At the very minimum, rooms for communal use should have links to the outdoors, which is of course what many people will have been used to in their own homes if they had an outside space.

Communal rooms

Living and dining areas that have doors to outdoor spaces can become much more lively and useful rooms. In good weather, the doors can be opened and fresh air, outdoor sounds and sunshine can flow in. Activities can spill outside where being tidy is not an issue, just like home. The door must be clearly visible and easy to open, while the outside surfacing needs to be 'barrier free' with no changes in level, tone or texture which can create visuoperceptual issues.

'In-between' spaces

In more temperate regions such as northern Europe, there is often pressure to shut the door due to draughts, so having an 'in-between' space can be a great advantage. Such spaces might include a lobby or porch, sunlounge, conservatory, verandah and boot room.

Verandahs and decks are very common in warmer regions, such as southern UK, Europe, Australia and parts of the US, as they provide much needed shade and protection from the sun.

More widely, 'in-between' spaces may also include external covered spaces such as gazebos, geodesic domes or sheds. Spaces

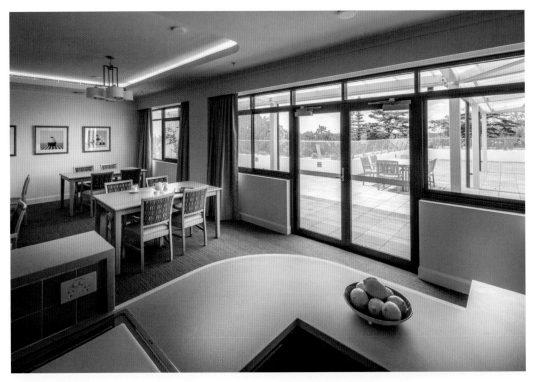

Access outside from the kitchen/dining room, HammondCare Wahroonga.

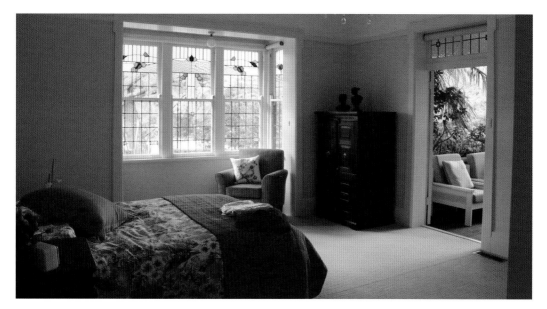

Access outside from a bedroom.

such as these provide somewhere to sit without actually being outside—the halfway house! They also provide a space where outdoor clothes and shoes can be stored as well as gardening equipment.

Another advantage of 'in-between' spaces is that they also allow the older eye to readjust to changes in light levels between inside and outside—but higher levels of artificial light inside the building may be required to help this.

Bedrooms

There are mixed views as to whether bedrooms should have direct access to the outdoors. This will depend on how the care home is managed—and also if the bedroom has a private sitting space as in a studio flat.

Key issues for discussion are:

- wayfinding—whether each resident can find his/her room with ease when coming back inside

- the capacity of the individual to cope with their own access out and finding their way back in

- ease of staff supervision of the outdoor space.

One way to make access flexible is to design the door from the bedroom to the outside so that it can be easily transformed in appearance to a simple window rather than a door. This allows access to be tailored to the needs of the resident.

Other rooms

Other rooms that can benefit from outdoor access are:

- activity rooms (activities are discussed in greater detail in Chapter 5)

- cafés

- laundry rooms for use by the residents.

Key points

- Many common design issues relating to accessing outdoors may present subtle barriers for people with dementia. However, these may be easily solved by thoughtful design.

- Weather is a key deterrent to going outside for many older people and people with dementia. Simple measures such as providing shelter and a choice of sun or shade can help.

- Create direct access from communal rooms wherever possible, as this allows activities to spill outside in good weather.

- Remember that 'in-between' spaces provide shade and shelter and are also places to prepare for exiting and re-entering the building.

- Consider the provision of outdoor access from bedrooms—but this may need careful management.

Opposite: A safe and inviting garden, Cairdean Nursing Home, Care UK, Edinburgh, Scotland. Photo: Annie Pollock

06
SAFE AND INVITING
'ROOMS OUTSIDE'

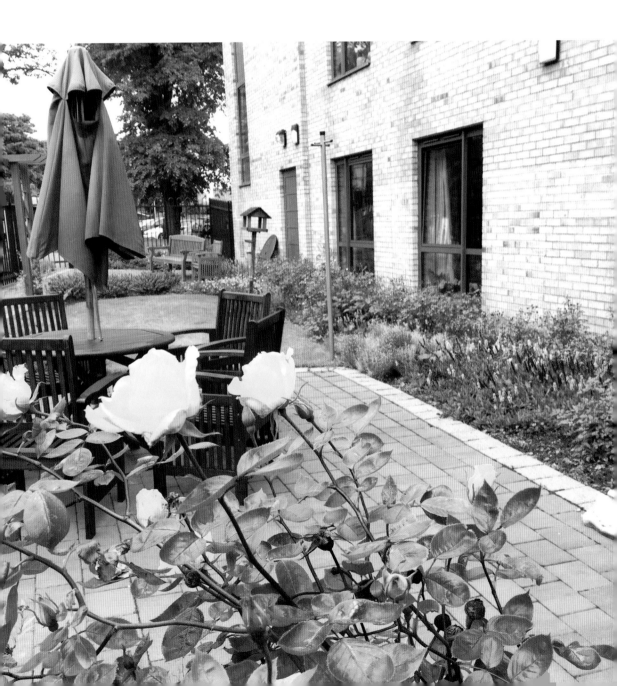

Outdoor areas for people with dementia must be safe. The design must also be familiar and inviting to encourage people outside. The following key elements need particular consideration.

Appropriate enclosure

The design of enclosing elements—including fences, walls, railings, gates and balustrades—will vary according to the country, its culture and the needs of the residents and staff.

In the UK, high fences or walls can seem imprisoning. Their design may vary according to the region of our small but varied country and it is worth seeing what is commonplace in the local area as this is likely to be more familiar to people with dementia. General recommendations are to:

- keep the enclosure as low as is safe to prevent unsafe exiting

- ensure that enclosures cannot be climbed—for example with timber palisade fencing, the horizontal rails should be on the outside where they will not provide a foothold. If, for reasons of external security the rails have to be on the inside face of the fencing, they should be triangular in section with paling attached to the flat side (so avoiding an easy foothold), or the fence could be double sided

- disguise the fence with planting to soften its appearance

- consider its colour— while there are no formal studies to verify this, dark green fencing in the UK has been reported to reduce attempts to exit.

From left: High fencing with climbers, Midpark Hospital, Acute Mental Health Unit, Dumfries and Galloway, Scotland. Low enclosure, Ferryfield House, Edinburgh, Scotland. Photos: Annie Pollock

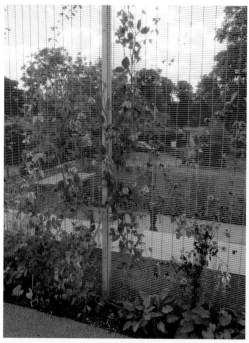 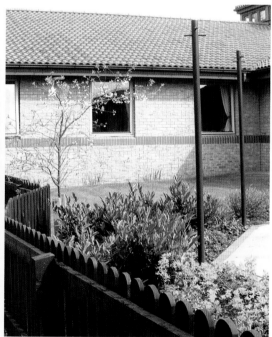

In Australia, higher, more visible enclosures around gardens and yards are common. Enclosures such as fences are accepted as boundary markers or for preventing people or animals entering your home and so are usually acceptable, even when quite high and visible. Even so, designing the fences so they are not unduly prominent is preferable.

Courtyards are a safe, secure and popular solution. In hotter areas of the world they provide a private and shaded open space for outdoor living.

However, in the northern hemisphere, courtyard dimensions need to be carefully considered against the height of the enclosing building to ensure sufficient sun penetration.

Camouflaging gates

Gates, which are not intended for use by people with dementia (as with doors for staff-only use inside the building), should be disguised or camouflaged. Locked doors or gates will promote frustration and distress in people with dementia. This means:

- making them look like a continuation of the fencing

- avoiding obvious handles or locks

- using mechanisms that require two-handed operation, while still being discreet

- colouring the path leading to gates in a different tone to deter the person with dementia from going that way

- using planting to disguise the way to these paths and gates where appropriate.

'The design of enclosing elements... will vary according to the country, its culture and the needs of the residents and staff.'

Balustrades on upper levels[48]

Multi-storey buildings with open spaces such as balconies or terraces have some special considerations.

Balustrades must be designed to prevent climbing while still facilitating direct sun access. For example, a balustrade could be designed to lean backwards into the balcony or terrace, which is hard to climb, however, this will reduce the usable floor area. Another solution is to have a planter on top of the balustrade, which inhibits climbing.

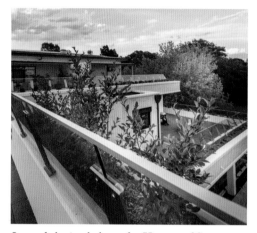

Inward sloping balustrade, HammondCare, Wahroonga, Australia.

High, glazed balustrades are often preferred as these allow people to see out and allow light through. But, as noted in Chapter 2, UVB rays, an important source of vitamin D, cannot pass through glazing. As we are designing for older people, and vitamin D is essential in maintaining their health, glazed balustrades must be low enough to allow direct sun access.

Deep balconies/terraces allow more sun access as higher balustrading will relatively affect less floor area—however, it is always worth checking at early design stages how much sun access you might expect throughout the year.

Surfaces that are enabling

Types of path surfacing will vary country to country although the general design principles remain the same. Some things can unsettle or be hazardous to the person with dementia:

- Changes in tone between the indoor and outdoor surfaces can look like a step or change in level, so ensure that internal and external surfaces have a very similar light reflectance value (LRV)—less than five.

- Changes in the tone (LRV) of abutting paved surfaces outdoors should be avoided too. However, to discourage a person with dementia from taking a particular path (e.g. a path leading to a gate for maintenance use), a strong change in tone can be effective.

- Avoid wide drainage channels with a shiny or coloured grid just outside doors to outdoor spaces. These can also look like a change in level—a slot drain will be a much less obvious solution.

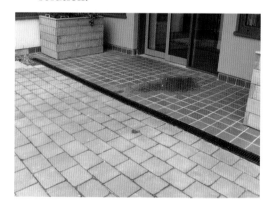

The black drainage channel could be seen as a change in level or step. Photo: Annie Pollock

- For people with visuoperceptual issues, visible joints in paving or patterned paving can be problematic.

- Light-coloured path surfaces can temporarily blind someone in bright sunlight. This is more common in sunny countries and with the use of white or light-tinted concrete surfacing.

- Service covers in a path can look like a hole or a patch of earth as they are nearly always a dark tone. It is better to use a recessed cover into which the paving material is inserted, as this will 'disguise/hide' the cover.

- Some patterned surfacing can look uneven and so are unsafe for older people or someone with dementia.

- 'Riven' slabs may trap puddles of water which could freeze over in cold climates or confuse someone with reflections, so are best avoided.

- Soft or gravelly finishes are difficult for wheelchairs, walking frames or for people who walk with a shuffling gait, so should also be avoided.

- Timber decking can become very slippery in wet climates, requiring regular maintenance. Composite decking is better, but can still be slippery.

- Rubber safety surfacing is sometimes suggested to minimise damage from falling. It's not a surface that is familiar to older people and it feels strangely bouncy. Its colour range can be limiting too. It would only be appropriate if there was outdoor exercise or children's play equipment in the outdoor space.

- Resin-bonded and resin-bound gravel are commonly considered surfaces.

Safe Surfacing

Aim for about 30% hard surfacing to 70% soft (grass/planting beds) – helps microclimate

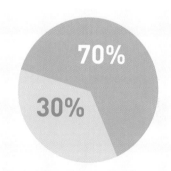

Generally suitable

- Block pavers
- Resin bound gravel
- Coloured asphalt
- paving slabs (small units better than large
- Concrete (in dryer climates)
- Decking (with care

Problematic

- Light/reflective materials
- Deeply riven slabs
- Very visible joints
- Loose gravel
- Bark mulch
- Safetly surface

Resin-bonded gravel is non-porous and may have some loose aggregate in the finish, which is less acceptable for people using wheelchairs or walking frames. Resin-bound gravel is a porous, smooth surface with no loose stones, providing a better and more sustainable finish. Care needs to be taken with the choice of aggregate, as some may be too speckled and/or too sharp in texture.

Trip hazards

It's important to remove trip hazards. Sharp corners to paths and raised edges are not advisable. A contrasting edge to a path can help people see where the path is going, but this should be flush with adjoining grass and planting beds to avoid a trip hazard, especially where the path turns a corner. The contrast edging must not run across paths where there are junctions as this could look like a change in level—which could cause falls.

Plant pots sited along a path can provide colour and look attractive—but they must be large enough to be clearly visible or they too could cause trips and falls.

Helpful handrails

In the UK and Australia, where there is a pathway with a gradient greater than 1:20, a handrail is required. This should be smooth and comfortable to use. In countries where the winter weather is very cold or the summer weather very hot, hardwood handrails are more forgiving than metal, as wood will get neither as cold or as hot as metal. To ensure it is clearly visible, the handrail should contrast against the ground surface and ideally the handrail supports.

Clear signs

Returning 'home' (which usually means finding the door to a familiar indoor living room or a person's own bedroom) should be possible to manage with little or no signage if everything is clearly identifiable and wayfinding is simple. The building, however, may have a complex layout, which will reflect on the garden layouts outside. There may be several different outdoor areas housing different things, such as a shed, garage, greenhouse, veggie patch, pond—and even items of memorabilia such as an old car (which many people may enjoy sitting in with memories of the Sunday drives they used to have).

Signage is a recognised part of the outdoor environment especially in towns and cities and may be very familiar to many people with dementia. With increasingly multicultural societies, a picture as well as lettering, is important for clarity. This will also useful for people with dementia who may find reading difficult. Text should be upper and lower case in a clear and uncomplicated font that is large enough to be clearly seen. Signs should be lower than might be considered normal, as older people can find it very difficult to raise their heads and look upwards.

Perhaps one of the most important signs should be to direct people outside to the nearest toilet, since the anxiety of this can be a strong disincentive to going outside in the first place!

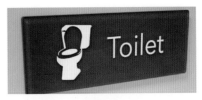

A clear and dignified toilet sign.
Photo: Mary Marshall

Places to sit, places to go

People who have reduced mobility may not venture outside at all if they cannot see places to sit. Ideally there should be plenty of seats, each one visible from the last to encourage walking. Choose seats which are sturdy but not so heavy that they cannot be moved to a better position. They should be comfortable, have arms to make getting up and down easy and be clearly visible against the ground.

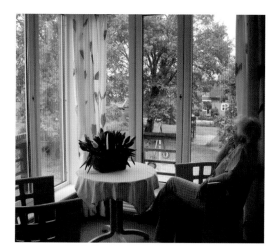

Good visibility

There are many advantages to having good visibility from inside the building to the outdoor spaces and vice versa. These include:

- being able to see outdoors, which will encourage people to go out—curiosity is part of human nature

- staff and carers being happier for people to go outdoors because they can clearly observe them

- known benefits to health and well-being from having a view outside to nature, first noted in the seminal research study by Roger Ulrich.[49]

Left: Seating at corridor end, Norway.
Photo: Garuth Chalfont, Chalfont Design.
Below: Therapeutic view from hospital wards,
Khoo Teck Puat Hospital, Singapore.
Photo: Annie Pollock

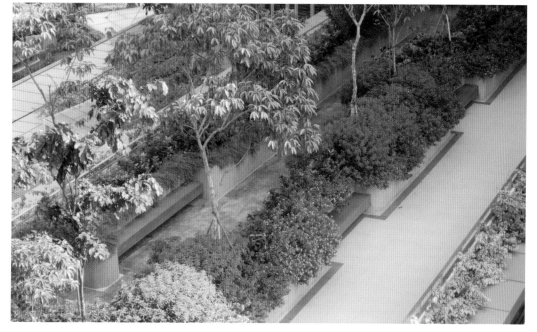

Key points

- Think safety and security, with both enclosure and gates.

- Ensure balustrading cannot be climbed but allows direct sunlight to the balcony or roof terrace.

- Carefully consider surface materials, tone, texture and jointing.

- Provide handrails and consider how they look and feel.

- Consider wayfinding and signage to ensure the person with dementia can find their way out, around the garden and back in again.

- Clearly indicate the nearest toilet.

- Have plenty of places to sit and rest and destinations to go to.

- Ensure good inter-visibility, from inside the building over the outside spaces and from outside, back to the door into the building.

- Keep in mind the need for tonal clarity, with more than 30 LRV between things that need to be seen and less than 5 LRV between adjoining surfacing.

- Remember the benefits of views of nature to health and wellbeing.

Well-designed outdoor seating, HammondCare, Erina, Australia.

07
FURNITURE AND STRUCTURES

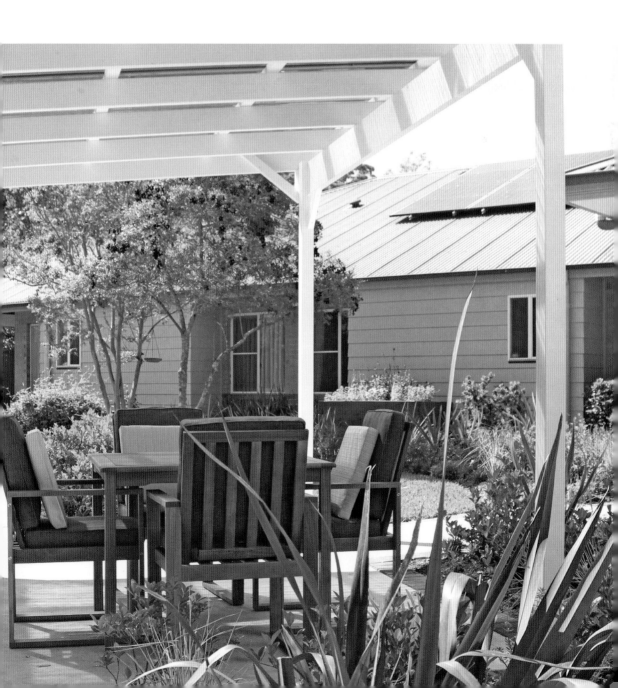

Outdoor areas for older people and people with dementia need more than just gardens and plants to be effective and enjoyable. A range of furniture is vital, so that people can sit outdoors. Items of interest that help initiate conversation, shade and shelter and things to encourage activity and stimulate memory are also important. All of these must be recognisable, safe and easy to use and clearly visible.

Seats and tables

As mentioned earlier, seating areas create a more inviting outdoor space. Having plenty of seating will encourage walking, particularly if between sitting areas there are places to go, destinations with things to do along the way and plants that are pleasant to walk past. If the next seat is clearly visible from the last one, this will encourage people to walk further.

The exact style of seat may vary country to country, but the same design parameters apply—seats must be stable, comfortable and easily seen. Remember that metal furniture can be cold or get too hot; plastic furniture can be too lightweight and easily toppled over; stone furniture can also be cold or hot and retain rainwater. Benches with timber slatted, rattan or woven seats are generally the most comfortable and sustainable.

Tables are vital for people to sit at, chat with a 'cuppa', play games, partake in a hobby, or simply read a book. Tables need to have enough legroom, particularly for people in wheelchairs. Square or round tables are better for people with dementia, as this enables them to see the person they are talking to, which is particularly helpful for people with hearing impairments. Larger tables may mean people sit side by side, which limits easy communication.

Square tables should have rounded corners to lessen the risk of injury.

Other features

Choosing planters

Raised planters of different heights enable people who are ambulant, as well as those in wheelchairs, to work at planting small plants and shrubs. Planters can either be built-in or mobile. Built-in planters are most useful as an 'allotment area', whereas mobile planters are useful for planting out seedlings or annuals and can be used on patio areas adjoining communal and activity spaces within the building. For those on a limited budget, planters can be made out of old pallets or woven willow. A planter designed to hold individual planting pods (e.g. Instaplanta in the UK or Vegepod in Australia or the US) makes for an even more flexible solution and can be easily moved if all the pods are taken out first.

Pergolas and trellises

Pergolas and trellises are used for training the growth of plants up and over. They can provide useful dividers between different areas, e.g. a veggie garden and a lawn and planting bed area.

Pergolas can be of any length—and in hotter climates can provide welcome shade once the planting has been established. The structure, however, before it is covered with plants (or roofing as may be the case in Australia), may cause confusing shadow patterns on the ground and so narrower structures may pose less of a problem in this respect.

Trellises are a useful backing to sitting areas, providing shelter and a feeling of security.

Bird tables, baths and feeders

Features that attract birds can provide lots of pleasure and interest to residents, but of course someone must take responsibility for keeping them clean and stocked. Staff may need to keep an eye on these, as some people with dementia may not understand the purpose of the bird food.

Structures that welcome

There are many outdoor structures that can provide a welcome destination point and seating area for people walking round the outdoor area. These include:

- gazebos
- arbours
- summerhouses
- geodesic domes.

There are many different garden buildings to choose from and climate may determine which are feasible. Any garden building should be:

- barrier free (i.e. no step up or down)
- clear for residents to see
- comfortable, with easy seating and room for at least two people
- in a location which allows for staff supervision.

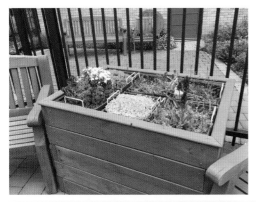

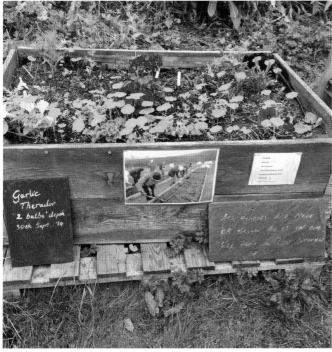

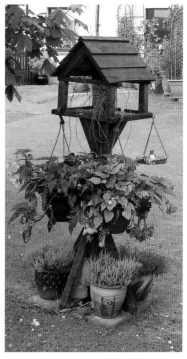

From top left: Instaplanta wth lift-out pods. Planter made of old timber pallets. Bird table in a retirement housing garden. Photos: Annie Pollock

More outdoor inclusions

Outdoor dining

Allow plenty of space for outdoor dining and a built-in barbecue—these can provide such fun on warm sunny days. This particularly applies in those countries where cooking and dining outdoors is part of the lifestyle and culture.

Buildings for meaningful activities

Sheds and greenhouses are the two most obvious buildings to offer meaningful engagement in an outdoor area, although there are other options. A care home in rural Australia for example, has an open, barn-like construction for a tractor and other farming equipment.

The Men's Shed movement in Australia and other countries is also regularly being incorporated into dementia care homes.

Ideally, all of these structures should be barrier free—this is easier with the greenhouse, but the garden shed might require a small ramp to make access easy—or a very clearly defined step and handrail too.

Allotments too!

If there is enough open space, a gardening allotment area can be provided for the more active residents.

An outdoor water tap is very useful, making it easy for residents to water plants. This may need to be done with supervision and the ability to lock the tap should be considered.

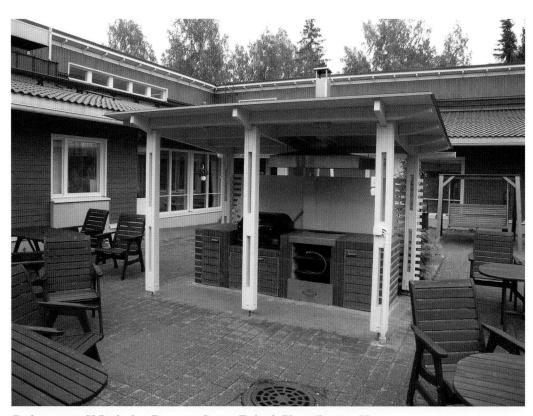

Barbecue area, Valkeakosken Dementia Centre, Finland. Photo: Damian Utton

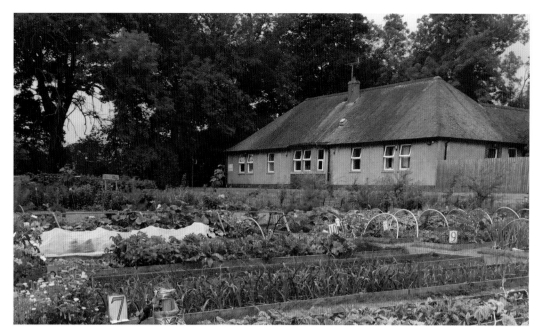

Allotment area, Cyrenians' Community Garden, Royal Edinburgh Hospital, Scotland. Photo: Annie Pollock

Water and recycling tanks

In many countries where water can be scarce (such as Australia), tanks for catching rainwater are common, particularly near farmhouses. Also, in many urban areas, water recycling tanks for gardens are increasingly mandatory. In one aged care home in the rural Hunter region of NSW, water tanks capturing rain from rooves feature in outdoor spaces. When one city visitor commented that it was not perhaps the most attractive view, the local older resident replied that it was what they had lived with all of their life and so was comforting in its familiarity![50]

In the south of the UK in particular, there have been bans on watering with hosepipes (garden hoses) in some years in the summer months—and with climate change this may become more usual. So a water butt for catching rainwater from the roof via downpipes is advisable.

Right: Outside toilet at Cowan Court, Penecuik, Scotland. Photo: Richard Pollock

Don't forget the toilet

Many older people grew up with outside toilets and are familiar with them. The great advantage of having a toilet outside is that people are more likely to go outdoors if they are confident getting to the toilet when they need to. It is recommended that the doors of toilets within a building should be a 'signature colour' and the outdoor toilet is no exception. Clear signage to it and on the door is useful.

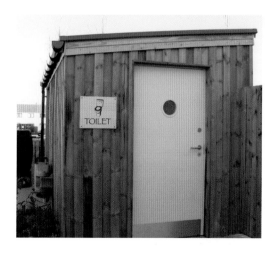

Case study 6
Clisham Ward, Western Isles Hospital, Scotland[51]

A special garden was created at the Clisham Ward of Western Isles Hospital, Stornaway for patients with dementia, to improve health and wellbeing, give a greater degree of independence and provide access to the outdoor world.

The garden enables people to go out at their leisure and enjoy the fresh air. It includes a sensory garden with a circular footpath and various features which help remembrance and reflection on aspects of past life and environment. A central feature is a geodesic dome (a Solardome® Haven, 4.5m diameter) which provides a warm, safe and quiet retreat and allows people to be in the outdoor environment in all types of weather. Being of circular design with curved benches, it affords good views of the wild flower meadow and shoreline dotted with lobster pots, and enables a closer social interaction for people with dementia and their carers.

Robert Stubbington, the Landscape Architect for the Western Isles Council (Comhairle nan Eilean Siar) said the Solardome® glasshouse was chosen because of its ability to be a unique focal point (which can aid wayfinding) and also because of its strength and longevity in the most extreme weather conditions. 'Our vision was to create a peaceful, tranquil environment for patients who are used to a natural way of life and who benefit from having access to natural light.'

The aim of the garden is to encourage patients to enjoy fresh air and exercise in a designed landscape, with increased feelings of wellbeing and reduced reliance on medication. The benefit of a dome such as this is that even in poor weather, patients may benefit from bright outdoor light which helps regulate their circadian rhythm.

'The aim of the garden is to encourage patients to enjoy fresh air and exercise in a designed landscape, with increased feelings of wellbeing and reduced reliance on medication.'

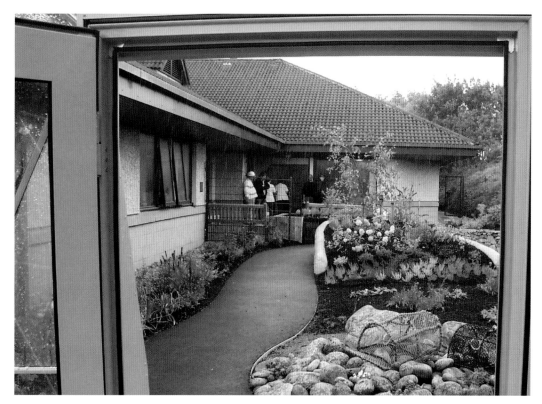

View from the Solardome, Western Isles, Scotland. Photo: Western Isles Council

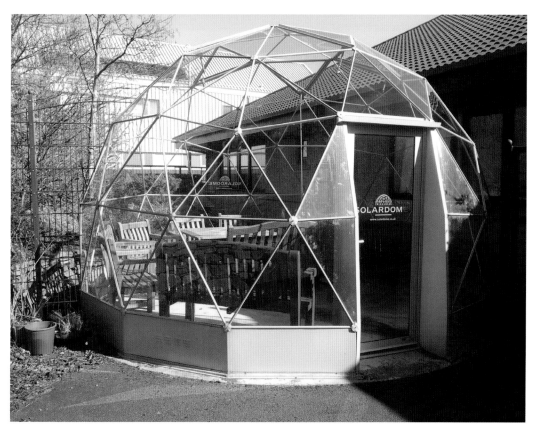

View of the Solardome from the garden. Photo: Solardome Industries

Key points

- Stable, familiar seating is vital for encouraging walking by providing a rest point.

- Smaller square or round tables allow for face-to-face conversation.

- Planters of varied heights and purpose make gardening more accessible.

- Pergolas and trellises with plants trained on them provide cover and screening (but be aware that large pergolas may cause confusing shadows due to the overhead beams).

- Structures such as gazebos and summerhouses provide welcome destination points.

- Familiar work areas such as sheds and greenhouses provide a common outdoor experience for many.

- An accessible outside toilet and a tap for watering are helpful additions to encourage people outdoors.

08
DESIGNING
WITH PLANTS

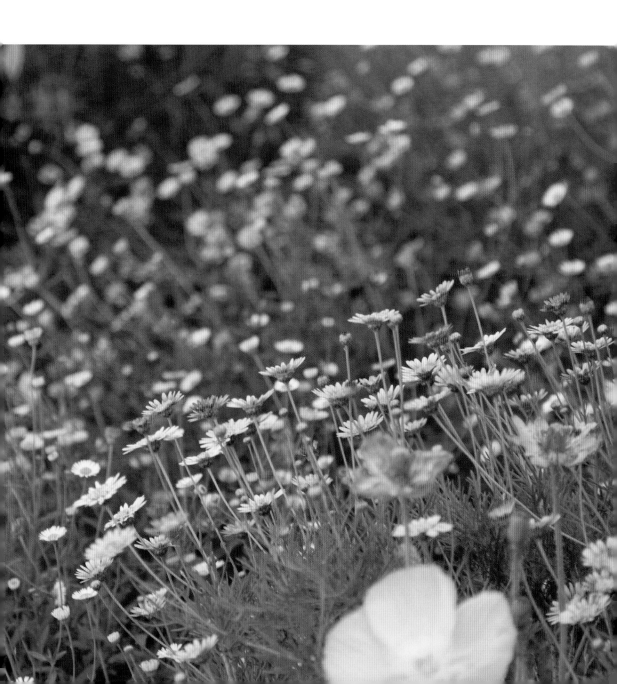

Plants not only 'furnish' the 'rooms' outside, but provide character, affect microclimate, and may have sensory attributes such as sound, touch and smell. Some plants can even help to reduce traffic pollution. The planting needs particularly careful design to be meaningful and familiar for older people and people with dementia.

During the design process, those who will maintain the garden should also be involved, so that they understand the design concept and can also contribute to it. Poor maintenance can ruin a garden in a very short time!

Plants that are meaningful

People may relate to plants that are not necessarily native, for example in the UK many garden plants are exotics, brought back by 18th and 19th century explorers. Many Australians love plants that they remember from their home countries—e.g. the UK, mainland Europe or parts of Asia.

So, finding a spot for the plants that the people you are designing for hold dear in their memories is always a good idea.

Selecting the right plants.

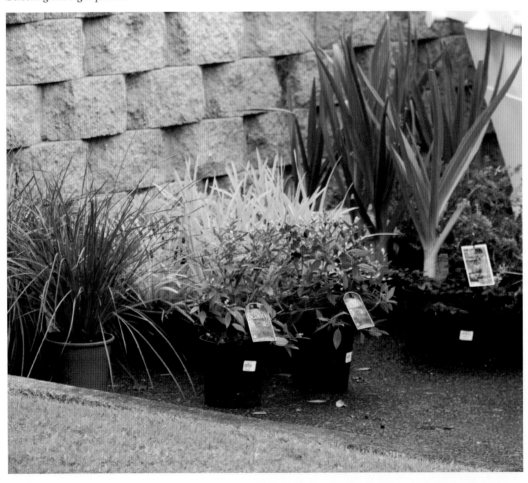

Microclimate matters

Plants need to thrive, by being well adapted to the climate and soil of the area, with sunshine, adequate water and maintenance. Consider the following:

- What plants grow well in the local area?

- Does the site itself have a particular microclimate which is different to the surrounding area (e.g. due to local landform)?

- Are the outdoor spaces exposed to the prevailing winds? If so, consider how best to provide shelter with planting, screens, trellises etc.

- Is there sufficient shade, or too much?

- If near the coast, are the outdoor spaces affected by salt spray? This can influence the type of plants that will thrive.

Planting design

Perhaps the important thing to consider at the beginning of any design is to work out the basic structure and concept of the garden, creating a framework in which plants can be moved about over the years or additional plants can be added.

Getting expert design and planting advice is vital—use an appropriately trained person who knows about plants and planting. It's too easy to make mistakes if you are not an expert, for example, there may be many cultivars of a particular plant which can vary from dwarf (c. 500 mm height and spread) to large (c. 1.5 m high or more), yet the generic name is the same. Detailed knowledge is vital to avoid getting the wrong plant in the wrong place!

Clients often say they want a 'maintenance free garden'—there is no such thing—although some plants need less care than others. Using ground-covering plants, however, does help prevent unwanted weed growth, so knowing the right plants to minimise hard weeding work will again need expert advice.

Stretching your plant budget

If funds are tight, you could consider creating a 'wish list'—a list of plants that would be ideal within the basic design framework. Many relatives like to make a gift to facilities where a member of their family has lived or been cared for and giving plants to help furnish a garden could be such an opportunity. A 'wish list', will also help you achieve a coherent design.

Growing your own

While on the topic of how to resource your planting, having a greenhouse and someone with 'green fingers' can be very useful. Many plants can be propagated from cuttings and this can provide a useful activity for residents.

The greenhouse and/or planters can also be used to propagate vegetable seedlings for the allotment, where space allows for one.

What kind of plants are appropriate?

Safe and non-toxic

People with dementia may want to handle, touch and even taste plants, so the plants must be safe in all respects.

Edible plants can provide a wealth of interest and activity, stimulate memories and, most importantly, stimulate appetite. Perhaps residents can be involved in harvesting plants for use in the kitchen. This could also result in a 'harvest festival' celebration and a 'thanksgiving' opportunity, which many residents may enjoy. Vegetable plots can provide welcome activity for the more physically able and planters for those who are less able.

Both flowering and fruiting plants give residents the opportunity to cut or pick flowers and fruit to bring indoors. This provides a connection with seasonal change.

Some garden plants are poisonous, for example *Laburnum*, the seeds of which can kill. Most botanic gardens can advise on this and there is a wealth of information on the Internet.

Finally, some plants may be prickly, the sap may be an irritant, the leaves may be sharp or spiky—so good research is required.

Below: Herbs provide sensory interest and are also edible!
Opposite: Japanese maple with shape, form, year-round interest and cultural significance too.
Photo: Annie Pollock

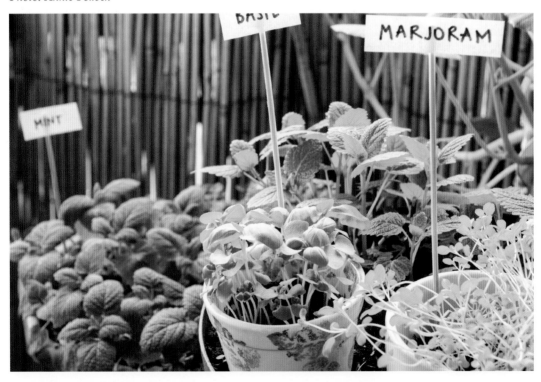

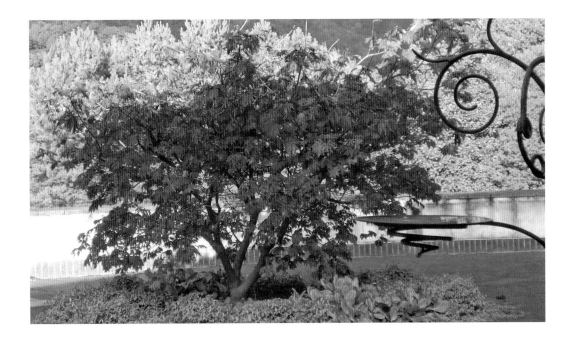

Sensory interest

Colour, touch, sound, scent and taste—these are all important attributes for people whose senses are generally diminishing.

It is important, however, not to have too many plants with sensory attributes—as there is the risk of causing confusion.

Many such plants also attract wildlife which can provide interest and activity, such as residents keeping a note of all the birds, butterflies and insects spotted in the garden.

Shape and form

Plants that have an interesting shape, colour of leaves or bark and are recognisable whatever the weather, can be particularly useful in wayfinding—as well as providing an attractive view from within the building. These are the building blocks of your design!

Year-round interest

Gardens need to look good whatever the season and plants which show seasonal change help the person with dementia relate to the passing of time, spring to winter.

Local or cultural significance

Some plants may have particular importance for the person with dementia, because they belong to the locality, are significant in their cultural or religious life or remind them of where they were brought up.

How about a gardening club?

Setting up a gardening club can encourage interest and participation. A Scottish housing association, providing sheltered housing for older residents, did just this—and also had an annual competition for the best results. Interest was enormous and competition stimulated conversation, cooperation and most importantly, activity!

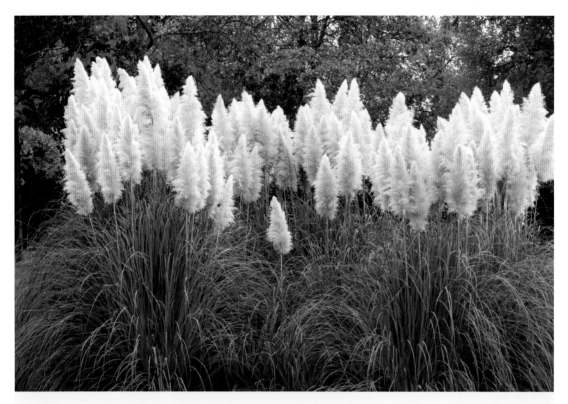

Pampas Grass. Beautiful plant, but can become hard to live with!

Case study 7
Good ideas with unintended consequences

A developer sought advice on his landscape architect's scheme as to its suitability for people with dementia. One plant specified was 'hops' (*Humulus lupulus*)—perhaps because it was a local plant. On further investigation, it was found to cause dermatitis in some people, so it was best avoided!

Another scheme proposed planting a block of 12 pampas grass plants (*Cortaderia selloana*). These are normally planted as one specimen as they can become very large—but in any case, the leaves have very sharp edges and are potentially harmful to someone touching or falling against them (and are now considered a noxious weed in some countries, such as Australia, where they self-seed prolifically). Again, best avoided.

These examples show the importance of checking the safety of all plants used, particularly those that are in accessible locations.

Key points

- Ensure there are sunny areas for the planting beds.

- Provide good, knowledgeable maintenance.

- Use only non-harmful plants.

- Use plants of local, cultural significance—plants that stimulate memory.

- Ensure that there are some edible plants such as fruit, vegetables and herbs.

- Design a planting scheme to provide year round interest.

- Consider clubs for outdoor activities.

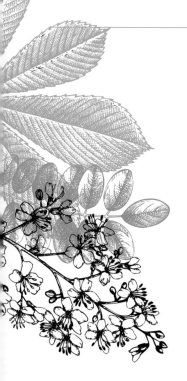

'Plants not only "furnish" the "rooms" outside, but provide character, affect microclimate, and may have sensory attributes such as sound, touch and smell.'

09
THE USE OF
LIGHT AND WATER

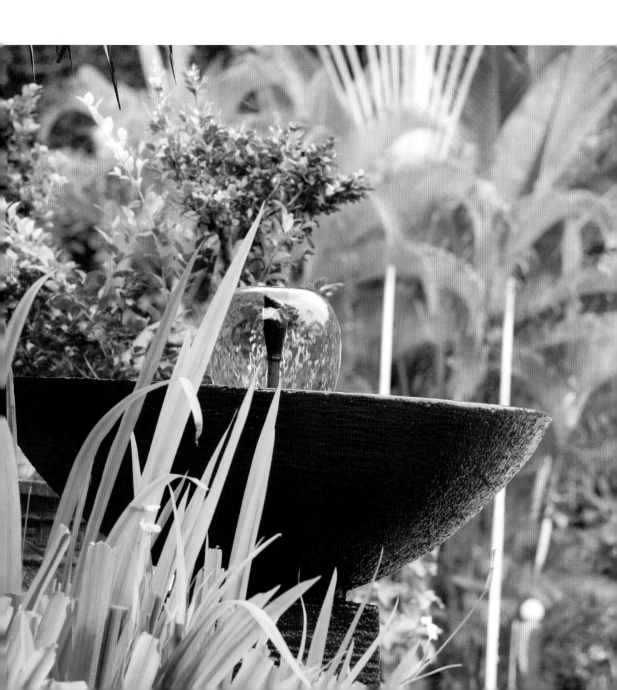

The value of lighting

Some of us like to go to bed early while others are 'night owls' and appreciate going outdoors after dark to see the night sky and enjoy the evening quiet and coolness (weather allowing!). Sometimes too, evening outdoor events may be organised, and for these and other reasons, outdoor lighting is indeed very useful.

When residents have finished using outdoor spaces in the evening, it is preferable that outdoor lighting is turned off or down (to security levels) either through automatic movement sensors, timers or manually by staff or carers. The exact timings for managing lighting levels should be determined by latitude, season and the operation of the individual facility.

Where to place the lighting

To achieve an even spread of lighting over the outdoor areas, it is best to mount the light fittings at a reasonable height. In its design, consider:

- ease of maintenance access which must of course be in accordance with the health and safety regulations of the region or country concerned

- provision of a lighting and/or power source in any outdoor shelters or gazebos for evening activities.

Generally, building-mounted solutions are better than lighting columns, as they provide a good spread of light to external areas and are a more economic solution. The design needs to avoid upward light spill and their spacing should ensure that there are no shadow areas at ground level.

Where there are no buildings close enough to the outdoor areas requiring illumination, lighting columns are the best solution for a good spread of light. Light sources would typically be mounted at between 3-4 m height from ground level, depending on the specific requirements.

'People are usually attracted to well-lit features or areas—consider carefully what is highlighted!'

Types of light fittings

The type of lights will depend on the layout and features of the outdoor areas. The type of light fitting will then influence the number needed to effectively light the required area.

For areas of soft landscaping including a footpath, the best results are usually achieved using luminaires having a symmetrical distribution (circular). If lighting a path only, it is best to use a fitting with an asymmetrical distribution (rectangular), where the light output shines along the path with minimal light spill to either side.

Lighting columns should be of a traditional style, familiar to people with dementia. Very modern styles could be confusing and disturbing for people with dementia, who may not recognise them for what they are.

Building mounted fittings should have no upward light spill and their spacing should ensure that there are no shadow areas at ground level.

Illuminated bollards should not be used as the principal light source, as they do not give a good spread of light and can form pools of shadow, which could be very confusing for people with dementia. If they are to be used at all, (for example in car parking areas) care should be taken to ensure that they:

- do not emit upward light that causes glare

- are not placed where they could be a trip hazard

- are located where vehicles cannot damage them.

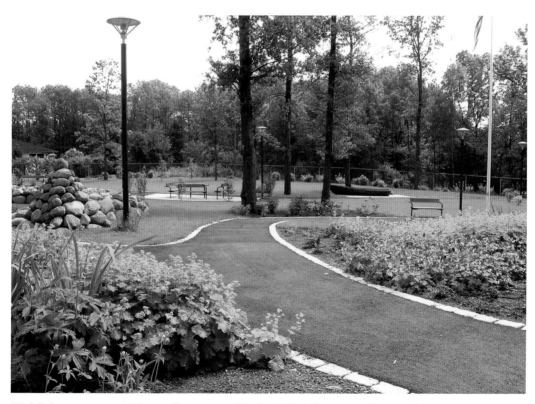

High light sources provide better illumination, Nes-Bo Behandlingssenter (living and treatment centre), Tonsborg, Norway. Photo: Damian Utton

Some bollards allow for the direction of light to be changed to suit conditions, and this could be helpful for ensuring a good spread of light cover over the footpaths at night.

Light fittings that are recessed into side walls, ramps or retaining walls can be helpful in wayfinding, but care must be taken to avoid glare or patterns of light which could be confusing.

Light fittings that are set into the ground surfacing are best avoided, as invariably there are failures due to water ingress. In addition, glare can be an issue. If low-mounted light fittings are to be used, it is best to install them on short brackets to achieve at least 250 mm above ground level, and be placed where they will not be a trip hazard, e.g. planting beds.

Fittings that last

Outdoor light fittings will need to withstand the elements. In the UK, for example, the minimum ingress protection rating of outdoor light fittings should be IP54 (where 5 = protection against dust ingress and 4 = protection against low pressure water ingress, such as splashing or rain).

In general, mild steel components (including lighting columns) should not be used outdoors unless they are protected against corrosion by hot dip galvanising.

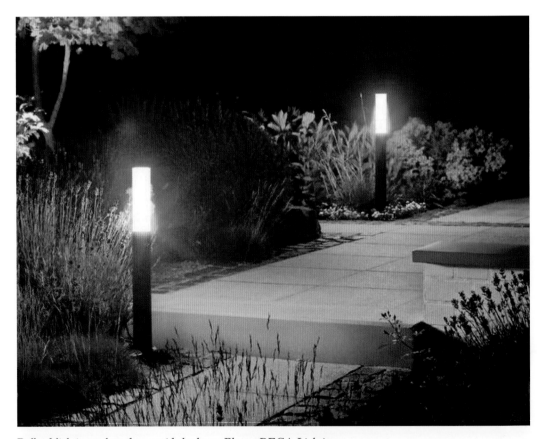

Bollard lighting, selected to avoid shadows. Photo: BEGA Lighting

Effects of lighting

People are usually attracted to well-lit features or areas, so consider carefully what is highlighted through lighting. Use lighting to draw people to safe and purposeful night-time outdoor areas. On the other hand, avoid highlighting features that are better used during the day, for example, water features. If it is still possible, however, for people to stray into them, the ambient lighting should be sufficient to allow the area to be easily seen from both inside or outside the building.

Light pollution

Lighting can lead to unwanted light intrusion or pollution, so it is important to consider the light spread of proposed fittings carefully by:

- choosing fittings that avoid upward light spill which can pollute the sky

- accounting for the location of street lighting in respect of bedrooms—many people will find external bright lights will seriously disturb their sleep

- providing black-out blinds as required.

Lighting advice

Always consult a lighting engineer to get an appropriate lighting design for outdoor areas. The engineer will be able to advise on suitable light fittings and lighting levels for different situation such as:

- stairs and ramps

- areas immediately around seats and benches

- pathways

- features that are appropriate to highlight

- night-time security.

And consult our companion book on lighting, *Enlighten*, which has comprehensive lighting advice for all aspects of dementia design.

What about water features?

We are often asked about the value of including water features in outdoor spaces for people with dementia. Water is an important aspect of garden design in several world faiths and this is discussed in Chapter 10 'Cultural and spiritual considerations'. People generally love water—it provides movement to look at, often a very pleasing sound and, of course, the sensory enjoyment of dabbling fingers in the water.

Water feature that provides interest and is safe for people with dementia, Uplands Sensory Garden, Shrewsbury, England. Photo: Marches Care Ltd

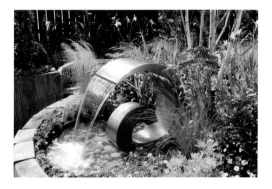

Important considerations

If including a water feature, the following factors are essential:

- Locate the water feature in a sunny area—shady areas under trees can mean lots of maintenance to keep the water fresh and free of debris.

- Ensure the design is meaningful— the cultural background of the people for whom you are designing will have a big part to play in formulating a design.

- The water feature must be safe for everyone. Ideally a person can visit on their own, for the peace and spiritual contemplation that it may provide. Children too will visit and their natural inquisitiveness must be taken into account to avoid any accidents— small children can drown in only 50 mm of water.

- Consider the sounds made by the water feature—not all are appropriate, with some sounding like slapping canvas, others like being in a toilet cubicle. It is important to listen to the working fountain or water feature before making an investment. A pleasant sound of water can also be useful in masking less attractive sounds on the site, such as traffic.

- Think carefully about how much space the water feature will occupy. One care home in Scotland accepted a gift of a pond and bridge in their courtyard from a relative of one of their residents. It was later decided that it took up far too much usable space. This decision was made with consideration of how much the pond and bridge contributed to the wellbeing of the residents.

- Regular and thorough maintenance is essential and it's important to meet your local infection-control officer to agree with what is necessary.

- Where water is not appropriate, artwork may be an alternative (see photo).

'People generally love water—it provides movement to look at, often a very pleasing sound and, of course, the sensory enjoyment of dabbling fingers in the water.'

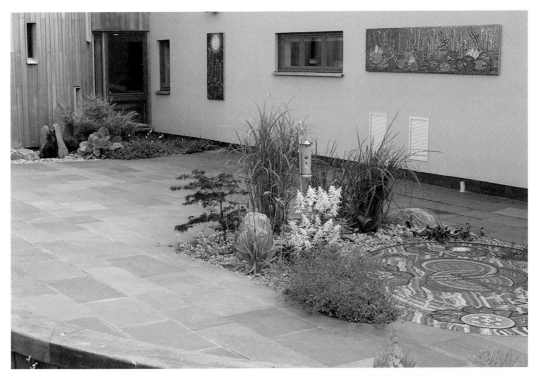

An attractive alternative to real water: Robin House Hospice, Balloch – Children's Hospice Association Scotland. Photo: Annie Pollock

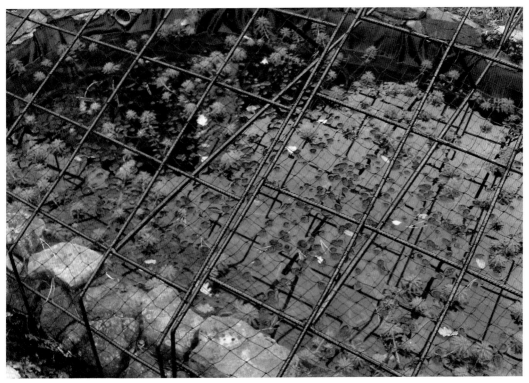

A safe water feature, Mowat Court Care Home, Care UK, Stonehaven, Scotland. Photo: Richard Pollock

Key points

Lighting

- Appropriate lighting supports outdoor activity at night.

- Ensure an even spread of light, avoiding shadows and glare.

- Choose traditional-style light fittings that people with dementia will find recognisable or familiar.

- Consider carefully the reasons for, and possible effects of, highlighting outdoor features.

- Minimise light pollution, especially upwards to the night sky.

- Consult a lighting engineer.

Water features

- Water has spiritual significance for many people.

- The sights, sounds and feeling of moving water can be pleasant.

- Water can provide cooling in hot weather.

- Check the sound of a water feature before purchase.

- Ensure the design of the feature is meaningful to people with dementia.

- Consider safety of residents and children alike.

- Ensure that the water feature does not take up useful space at the expense of activities in the outdoor area. And regular maintenance is essential!

Opposite: Suburban style care home, St Catherine's View Care Home, Colten Care, Winchester, England. Photo: Annie Pollock

10
CULTURAL AND SPIRITUAL CONSIDERATIONS

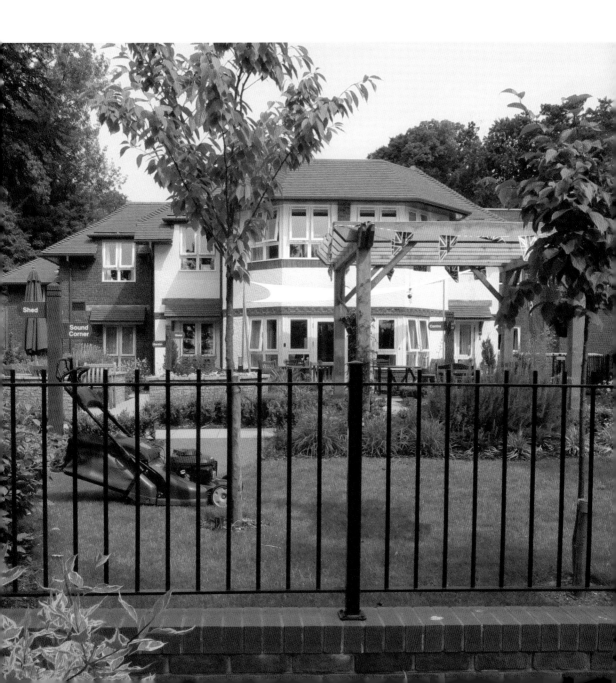

We live in a time when diverse cultures are increasingly found together in communities and care environments. When designing buildings and outdoor spaces for older people and people with dementia, we need to consider who is going to use the outside space. Here are some questions to ask:

- Where did the person grow up and what is familiar to him/her?

- Is the person from an urban, suburban or rural background?

- Does the resident's background and upbringing have gender traditions?

- Is there an episode in their life for which an area of 'commemoration' might be appropriate? This will require careful thought, discussion and management.

- Does the person have any religious preferences? Will they affect their use of outdoor spaces?

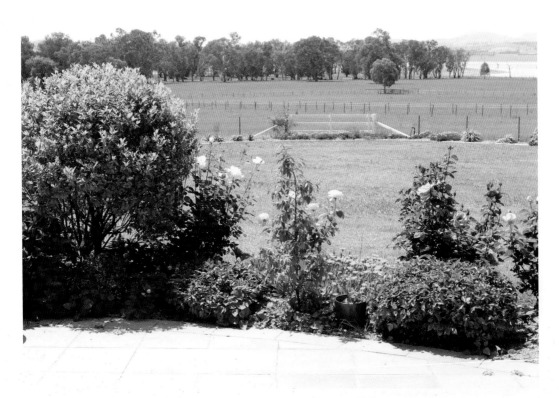

A rural setting

Focusing on the familiar

If, due to dementia, a person's recent memory has diminished, they will tend to make sense of a space in terms of their past.

One way of looking at this is to imagine people with dementia may be seeing the world through a different lens, perhaps from more than 60 years ago. It is also important to note, that what might be familiar to one person may not be to another. As an example, being outdoors will probably mean something very different to Indigenous Australians or North Americans than it does for those whose forebears came from Europe or Asia.[52]

Another variable is that the person now needing care may have spent their younger years in a very different place or country. Although migration has reached exceptional levels at present, it has always existed. For example, in the 1930s, huge numbers of people returned from the colonies to the UK and in the 1950s, huge numbers of British people went to Australia on the £10 fare. There have been waves of migration from all over the world to other countries.

People assimilate to varying degrees, but if their understanding of the present diminishes, they will have a greater reliance on the past to make sense of the world—and this may mean that their current environment becomes quite unfamiliar to them. This challenge increases if a person, due to dementia, reverts to using their mother tongue—different to the main language of their adopted country.

Considering residents' background

In addition to migration, many people were not born in the cities where they now live. A United Nations report, in 2014[53] states that:

> Globally, more people live in urban areas than in rural areas, with 54% of the world's population residing in urban areas in 2014. In 1950, 30% of the world's population was urban, and by 2050, 66% of the world's population is projected to be urban.

This means that many older people who were born in the countryside have moved to the city.

City dwelling too has always had many variants. People either lived in:

- suburbs and will have had a garden
- small houses with tiny yards
- apartment blocks, which may have been very high and housed many hundreds of people.

We can see that what is familiar in terms of outside space will vary greatly.

For those who lived in the countryside all their lives, gardens may be less familiar than broader outside space for growing crops, mending nets, working in forests or rearing animals.

Gender-related experiences

Gender may be another design consideration. In some cultures, men may have used outside spaces very differently from women. They may be more familiar with sports fields, bowling greens and golf courses for example, whereas women may have preferred spaces for picnics and a children's playground. For women, the garden or yard may have been a place for hanging out washing or reading a book in the sun, while for men, the same area might be for tinkering with a bicycle or car, keeping animals such as pigeons or chickens and having a shed. This is not to stereotype genders—there will be wide variety—but common experiences will often be evident among men and women.

Commemorative spaces

In many cultures, outdoor spaces can be beneficial and meaningful to people for remembering those who were lost in war (especially the world wars) or other catastrophes. Careful research is needed to ensure that the design of the space is meaningful to the people with dementia who will visit it—while also being careful the memory does not cause stress and anxiety.

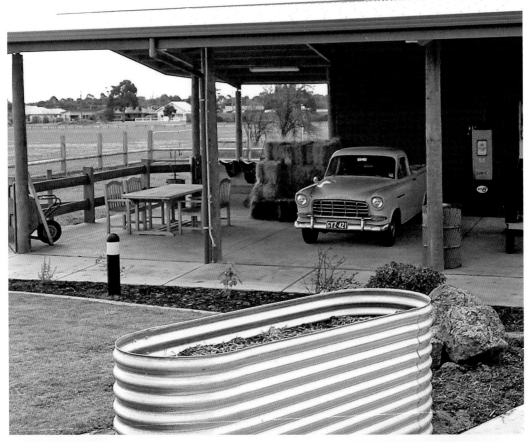

Utility shed in a rural care home, Hesse Rural Health Service, Winchelsea, Australia. Photo: Hesse Rural Health Service

Faith and spirituality

Religion, faith, spirituality—all can play a very important part in the design of outdoor spaces and the wellbeing of the residents because:

- all faiths need quiet spaces for contemplation

- some religions may have specific colours and plants that are important and meaningful, whereas for some very divided communities, colour can be a contentious issue

- water and its sound can have spiritual meaning.

It's important to be aware that if people don't belong to a specific faith and don't have any spiritual preference, they may still have cultural or individual preferences for the outdoor space. It's important to cater for each individual as far as possible.

The following information is only a snapshot of how outdoor spaces may look for some of the world's religions and faiths (listed in alphabetical order). More research is required if an outdoor resource for a particular faith is to be included in a care home designed for people with dementia. Research would also include talking with residents, families and spiritual leaders within the religion.

Baha'ism

For those of the Baha'i faith, the garden can be a reminder of the joyful nature of death:

- A long-lived tree (such as *Magnolia grandiflora* or *Gingko biloba*) could represent immortality—the bulb of a plant is like the enduring soul.

- Plants that bloom, die and grow again represent resurrection, e.g. snowdrops (*Galanthus*) and crocuses (*Crocus*) could symbolise the resurrection of spring from winter and the return of summer.

- The divine is readily symbolised by the sun, the Spirit by its rays.

- To people of the Baha'i faith—who see a perpetual succession of religions rising and falling and being renewed by the next—the seasons represent this rise and fall, with a perpetual process of renewal particularly at springtime.

- Springtime brings a new year for the Baha'i faith, held at the spring equinox.

- A small flow of water (done in a safe way) could represent the Spirit.

'It's important to cater for each individual as far as possible.'

Buddhism

Buddhism has the strongest connection to gardens of any world religion. It originated in the foothills of the Himalayas (c. 600 BC) and so it is understandable that mountains came to be associated with gods.

Buddhist gardens can be any size and will generally include paths for walking and seating areas for peaceful reflection, often under the shade of a graceful tree. Any unpleasant views, which might detract from the peaceful atmosphere of the garden, should be blocked with trellises or bamboo screens and climbing plants.

Fountains which produce a lovely sound and a pond with goldfish or koi carp are popular.

The Zen garden is the best known type of Buddhist garden and is designed with the principles of austerity (*koko*), simplicity (*kanso*), naturalness (*shizen*), subtlety (*yugen*), tranquillity (*seijaku*), imperfection and asymmetry (*wabi-sabi*).

A Buddhist garden may contain Buddhist images and art, but more importantly, it should be a simple, uncluttered space that reflects the principles above, together with respect for living things and the seasons.

Lanterns are a recognisable feature of Buddhist gardens, but their purpose isn't to provide light. They were originally used in temples and shrines as a sign of worship that honoured Buddha or revered ancestors.

Below is a list of plants that are meaningful for showing seasonal change (particularly in Japan).

- Cherry trees (*Prunus* varieties)—these signify the arrival of spring.

- Bamboo—some forms can be useful for the summer months, especially if the planting allows the sunshine to filter through the leaves. Bamboo needs to be chosen with care, as some forms are rather too aggressive.

- Japanese maple trees (*Acer* varieties), especially *palmatum* forms, come into their own in the autumn with bright coloured leaves. *Physalis* and *Cosmos* are popular too.

- Camellias (*Camellia* varieties) provide colour and interest in the winter months.

- *Nandina domestica* is a small, elegant evergreen shrub with an upright,

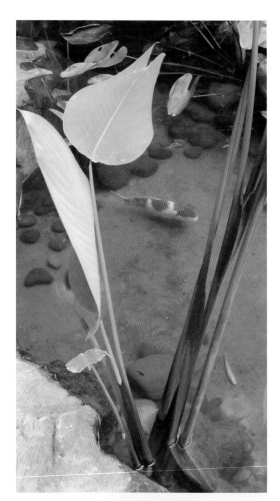

Koi carp, a popular Buddhist symbol in China and Japan. Photo: Annie Pollock

bamboo-like habit, purplish when young and again in winter. Small white flowers in large panicles are followed by red berries.

- Pines (*Pinus* varieties) are very popular, especially if they are shaped bonsai-style.

- The lotus flower (*Nelumbo nucifera*)—this is an important element in Buddhist garden design, respected for its ability to provide beautiful blooms even in shallow water.

Christianity

From God walking with Adam in the Garden of Eden to Jesus weeping in the Garden of Gethsemane, the garden in the Bible is a place full of spiritual significance. The role of nature itself as a pointer to God as a loving Creator is one that Christians hold dear. Being in a natural place to contemplate God's creation is also a key part of Christian meditation for many. The Christian scriptures are full of the symbols of rivers and water (thirsting after God, washing away sin, the bringing of joy). Jesus also references many parts of nature to explain what God the Father is like, for example 'Consider the lilies' and describes himself as 'the true vine' and his Father as 'the gardener'.[54]

In terms of designing outdoor spaces for Christians, a place for walking or sitting in quiet meditation amongst nature would most likely be welcome. There are also some symbols within the faith which could be incorporated within the detailed design, for example, the symbol of the fish (Ichthys), dove and cross would be well recognised.

Catholics may also appreciate images of the Virgin Mary or a crucifix as this is part of their tradition. Perhaps a small grotto or shrine in the garden area could also be considered.

Below is a list of plants which are symbolic within the Christian tradition.

- Apple (*Malus* sp.), when shown in Adam's hand, symbolises sin. When held by Christ, it represents salvation.

- Bulrush (*Typha* sp.) is used as a symbol of faithfulness and humility in obedience to Christ because the bulrush is a common plant that grows in clusters near water. Because of its association with the infant Moses, it may also point to the place of salvation (Exodus 2).

- Cedar of Lebanon (*Cedrus libani*) is a symbol of Christ. It is also identified with beauty and majesty.

- Grape vine—grapes represent the blood of Christ, especially in reference to the Eucharist. A vineyard represents the mission field, and grapes in this association may signify good works. A grape vine is a reference to Christ.

- Holly (*Ilex* varieties) is often used as symbol for Christ's crown of thorns, and therefore of His Passion.

- Sword lily (*Gladioli*) is a rival of the lily as a symbol for the Virgin Mary and refers to Mary's sorrow at Christ's Passion. However, the bulbs are poisonous and some parts of the plant can cause irritation so some care is needed with them.

- Ivy (*Hedera* varieties), being evergreen, represents faithfulness and eternal life.

- Lily (*Lilium* varieties) symbolises purity, the primary attribute of the Virgin Mary.

- Lily of the valley (*Convallaria majalis*) flower appears in early spring and so is often used to symbolise Christ's Advent.

- Olive (*Olea europaea*) trees are a universal symbol for peace and olive oil is a symbol of God's anointing and of the Holy Spirit.

- Palm—there are many varieties and climates and geographical relevance is likely to dictate whether this is appropriate. For many Christians, this is in remembrance of Christ's entry into Jerusalem on Palm Sunday, the palm representing a symbol of victory.

Hinduism

A typical Hindu garden is resplendent with beautiful tropical flowers, bright colours and sweet aromas. For example, the tulsi plant (*Ocimum basilicum*), a form of sacred basil, is important in the Hindu faith.

Orange is a special colour and traditionally, orange ribbons are tied on to tree branches at particular times of the year.

If translating the need for coloured and aromatic plants into a setting where the climate is cooler, then consider providing plants which have some of these attributes.

- Jasmine (*Jasminum* varieties) for perfume, montbretia (*Crocosmia*) for bright colour and the traditional marigold (*Tagetes* varieties) would be a good bedding out plant for planters and feature beds.

- A herb garden will provide smell, taste and stimulate culinary memories—and if climate allows, this might include basil too.

- Trees that have particular significance are the peepal tree (*Ficus religiosa*), the banyan tree (*Ficus benghalensis*), the ashoka tree (*Saraca asoca*), the paijaat

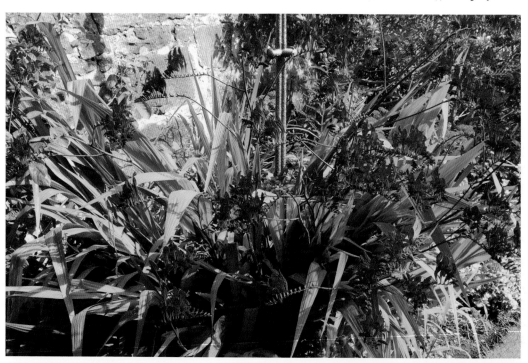

Crocosmia—Scarlet flowers are important for Hinduism. Photo: Annie Pollock

tree—which is a type of Baobab, and lastly, the sandalwood tree (*Santalum album*). Some of these would grow in the more tropical parts of Australia, but perhaps not in more temperate climates. However, hardy palms such as fan palm (*Chamaerops*), Chilean wine palm (*Jubaea*) and the chusan palm (*Trachycarpus*) are all types of trees common in hotter climates, but which can grow in cooler climates too.

Other features include trees that provide shade, walkways, water features and quiet places to sit and meditate.

Statues are not thought necessary, because for the Hindu person with dementia, nature herself is the great healer.

Islam

As with many gardens of faith, those for Muslims should generally be shaded and peaceful. Traditionally designed for rest and contemplation, they should include plenty of seating. The Ismaili Centre's garden in London is delineated by a central fountain and draws inspiration from the Qur'anic garden of paradise. Sheltered yet open, it combines granite and greenery with geometry, symbolism and the sound and flow of water. Visitors are treated to a sanctuary of calm amidst the bustle of the city below. Guests are greeted by scents of jasmine, lavender and herbs.[55]

The word 'paradise' is derived from the Persian word *faradis* meaning a place walked in. A typical Islamic garden is an enclosed space providing safety, coolness, shade, water, sweet scents, flowers and greenery. Grass lawns are not a characteristic feature of Middle Eastern gardens.[56] A courtyard, or at least a semi-enclosed design, is particularly appropriate for people with dementia of

Islamic faith. Also, consider some form of shelter against the elements outside—such as a canopy or gazebo.

The following pointers provide a guide to general design considerations:

- When a mosque is full on important religious occasions, the courtyard is used as an overspill space. Before praying (normally up to five times a day), Muslims must wash their hands, feet and over their head. This can be done at a pool or fountain and ideally in running water.

- It's important to have indication of east and west (depending on the location in the world) so as to work out the direction of the Qiblah for prayer. A simple and easily visible compass might be a feature within the space.

- Men and women may need separate spaces and women may prefer partitioned or secluded areas, to maintain their privacy and safety—this will depend on their upbringing and cultural background.

- Plenty of seating should be provided and these could be tiled to provide a familiar space. Whatever type of seating is provided, it should be safe and stable, with arms to help older people sit and rise up again.

- If the dementia is severe, specialist intervention may be required to help the individual recall some of the rituals e.g. pictorial depictions of the ablution and prayer rituals. On the other hand, figurative art is widely rejected in Islam and depictions of Muhammad are considered especially offensive.

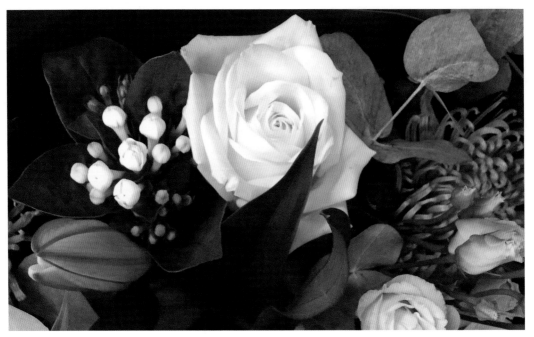

Roses are popular in the Islamic culture, due to their perfume. Photo: Annie Pollock

- Dogs are frequently noted as being helpful for people with dementia. However, many people of the Islamic faith see dogs as unclean and if touched by a dog's saliva, they must wash that part of their body. Consequently, many Muslims would rather not have contact with a dog—and this could be particularly problematic in outdoors, where animals are often more boisterous. Cats, however, are considered clean.

In terms of planting, remember that the garden is viewed as paradise. This means flowers, colours, perfumes and herbs, fruits and vegetables too—everything that Allah has provided. Date palms, if the climate allows, are particularly memorable, as dates are known as the food Muhammad ate when he broke his fast.

If there is an outside toilet (and this will also apply to toilets within the building), a facility for washing should be provided.

This might be a bidet, a spray fitting— or more simply a water vessel or 'Lota', a small round water pot, typically of polished brass.

Judaism

For Jews, a garden is a place for peaceful contemplation and meditation, a place where plants also provide meaning. Particularly important plants centre around the seven species listed in Deuteronomy 8:8, which include: wheat, barley, figs, grapevines, pomegranates, olives and date palm honey. Obviously many of these are climate dependent or impractical to grow in a small outdoor space, but the following are possible:

- Olive trees, grape vines and fig trees, which can survive quite well outdoors in more temperate climates.

- Some grasses might replicate the appearance of wheat and barley.

- Shrubs which have red leaves (e.g. *Pieris* varieties) or red autumn colouring (e.g. *Acer, Berberis* and *Cotinus* varieties) could represent the burning bush.

Once a year Jews celebrate the festival of Sukkoth (Feast of Tabernacles). This is an outdoor activity which involves the building of a temporary outdoor structure (a sukkah) e.g. a fruit adorned booth, partially open to the sky. If Jewish practice is to feature in a care environment for people with dementia and if there is enough outdoor space to do this, the means and support to build a sukkah would be very good for stimulating memory and activity. Alternatively, an outdoor gazebo or arbour which is permanently fixed in place, can also be decorated with fruit at the time of the festival by the residents.

Sikhism

A garden for people of the Sikh faith is a place for peace and relaxation. A water feature will provide comfort and familiarity to the person with dementia and their family—and most commonly this will include gently running water, lotus flowers and a bench under a tree. In the spring, marigolds (*Tagetes* sp.) are an important flower, representing Vaisakhi, which is a harvest festival of the Punjab region, celebrated in April. Some farming memories, e.g. a cart, or a sculpture of buffaloes, could bring back memories for many people who come from rural India. As marigolds are annual plants, it may be useful to have a raised bed or raised area for planting them out each year.

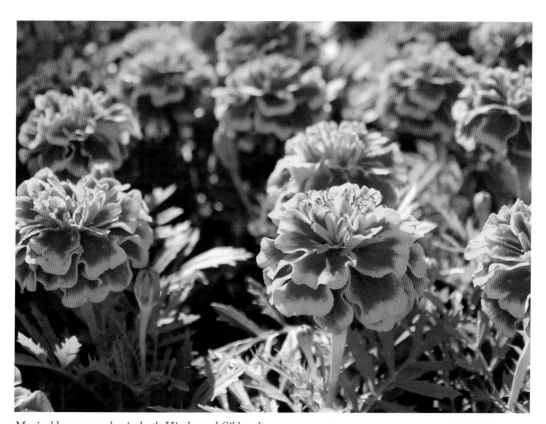

Marigolds are popular in both Hindu and Sikh cultures.

First peoples

Obviously, a wide range of people are covered by the terms First or Indigenous Peoples and it is not possible to make specific observations about outdoor spaces for them all. However, the needs of two well-known groups may offer broader insights and prompt further research.

Native American/Canadian[57]

Native Americans have a deep respect for nature. Ceremonies are the main way of religious expression and are normally held outdoors in contact with the earth.

The circle as a symbol, is sacred and the following directions and colours are also sacred:

- East (yellow)—usually the location of the spirit of enlightenment, guidance, and direction.

- South (black)—represents the spirit of growth, especially after the winter.

- West (red)—usually the doorway that one goes through when returning to the spirit world.

- North (white)—usually the location of the spirit of healing and reconciliation. These spirit helpers are always present and within the circle.

In addition, three other directions have significance: 'up' for Grandfather Sky, 'down' for Mother Earth and 'inward' for the heart.

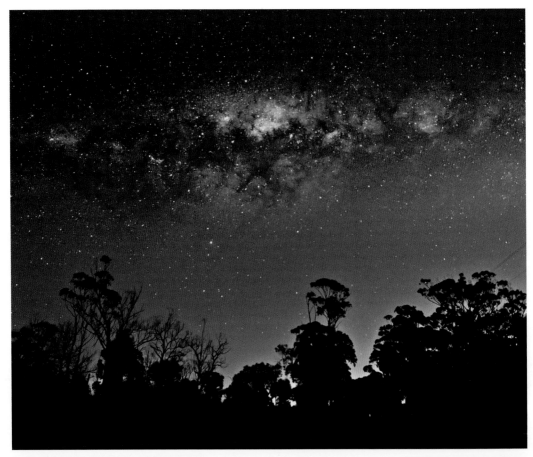

The night sky is integral to Aboriginal life.

The sweat lodge ceremony is particularly important. The lodge is a dome-shaped structure of willow or similar, lashed together with twine or bark, then covered with canvas or a tarpaulin to make it light-proof. A small pit is dug in the centre of the lodge in which rocks are placed. The doorway may face east or west according to the tribe. A small soft barrier is constructed around this area to protect it—this might be formed by a hedge or other plants.

If space allows, an area incorporating a sweat lodge could be constructed relatively easily, although attendance for people with dementia may need to be in supervised groups. If unable to incorporate the lodge, a circular motif in stones with a central stone hearth and associated planting could be built with seating for contemplation. Of course, care has to be taken that this does not pose any trip hazards. There are many tribes from very different areas and so consultation is essential to ensure that what is provided is suitable and correct.

Indigenous Australians

Aboriginal and Torres Strait Islander peoples—across many different language groups—have in common a deep spiritual sensitivity. This spirituality is strongly associated with the natural environment—land in all its forms, rivers, oceans, waterholes, trees, and wildlife. Particular landscape features as well as fauna and flora may recall stories of The Dreaming, which is often linked to creation. The land broadly—and to some extent—outdoor spaces, are *'food, our culture, our spirit and identity'.*[58] For many Aboriginal people, the location of a campsite or shelter, and in particular, the fire or hearth and its relationship to the mythological and physical landscape, carries symbolic meaning for a community's settlement pattern.[59]

Another aspect of Aboriginal life is the importance of the night sky. For more than 50,000 years, Aboriginal and Torres Strait Islander peoples have incorporated celestial events into their oral traditions and used the motions of celestial bodies for navigation, time-keeping, food economics, and social structure.[60] So, 'for many Aboriginal people, the sky has always been as much part of their world as the ground' and they traditionally used song and the stars in the sky to navigate and to tell them when to move camp.[61]

It is likely, then, that any outdoor spaces for Indigenous Australians would benefit from clear sky views to be comforting and to trigger memories of past times.

Other religions and beliefs

Accessibility to the outdoors and contact with the natural world is important for many other religions and beliefs. Ideally, there should be an area with plenty of available seating for events and a gazebo (permanent or a temporary tented structure) where participants and performers could gather—and with planting too, for a pleasant, soft and colourful environment.

How to meet different needs

The common notion that everyone appreciates and understands the various terms commonly applied to outdoor areas, such as 'sensory', therapeutic', 'healing' or 'spiritual' is probably not helpful for the diversity of backgrounds in care homes and hospitals. What appeals to the senses, provides therapy, healing or spiritual comfort for one cultural background may be unfamiliar to another. It is vital to understand your residents.

In many cultures, inner city dwellers will feel most at home in a park-like setting. Parks generally have a degree of formality about them, with paths, benches, flowerbeds and pavilions. Parks often have sports areas too and some recognition of this in the design of 'rooms outside' for people with dementia could be useful in providing for activity.

Suburban British people, however, would most likely feel more comfortable in a garden. Their counterparts in Australia would be used to having a yard with grass, a barbecue, shed and trees for shade.

For those from the countryside, outdoor spaces for working in a farming theme may be most familiar.

There may of course be people from many different backgrounds in one facility and so we need to consider what this means in design terms. It may well be necessary to provide a set of outdoor spaces.

'What appeals to the senses, provides therapy, healing or spiritual comfort for one cultural background may be unfamiliar to another. It is vital to understand your residents.'

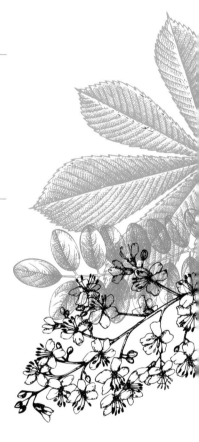

Case study 8
Domizil am Zoo—a care home in Dresden, Germany

Domizil am Zoo in Dresden, Germany, is a private care home managed by Axion Consulting Hamburg, providing 125 nursing care places and 50 dementia specific care places. There are also 30 apartments designed for older people to rent on the site. These tenants can also use the care home facilities.

The outdoor space at Domizil am Zoo is a great place to spend time with family and friends and features three traditional Bavarian water treatments developed by Sebastian Kneipp.

A showering area allows a person's knees to be 'doused' in water. A water-treading zone is for people to stroll through knee-deep cool water. Supposed benefits include better sleep, strengthened veins and a stimulated metabolism.

And then there is a high-level sink to complete the ritual by dipping elbows into cool, still water. The aim of the therapy is to stimulate circulation and all the senses. Proponents claim increased wellbeing, relaxation, stabilisation of body warmth, regulation of blood pressure, activation of immune system and ameliorated circulation of the skin.

Local children also visit and participate with the residents, adding to the enjoyment for all.

Also, there is a very shallow stream in the garden—the soothing sound of running water further enhances outdoor areas.

Together, these are highly appropriate activities for this care home—aside from any health benefits, they are familiar to residents, give brilliant sensory stimulation and the opportunity to connect with nature and other people in a fun and relaxed environment.[62]

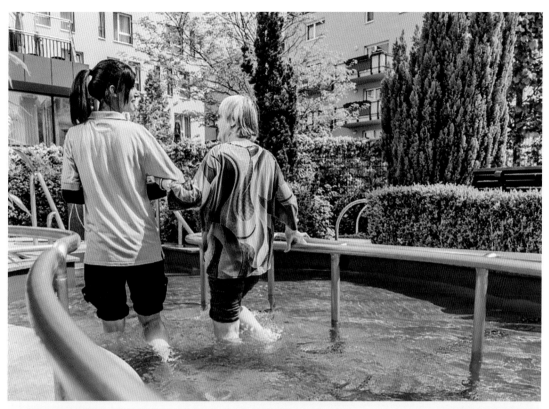

'Water-treading' as relaxation, Domizil am Zoo, Dresden, Germany.
Photo: Domizil am Zoo

'The outdoor space at Domizil am Zoo is a great place to spend time with family and friends and features three traditional Bavarian water treatments developed by Sebastian Kneipp.'

Key points

- Create an outdoor space that is familiar to the people with dementia who will use it.

- Understand and design for the cultural and religious background of the people with dementia and where they come from.

- Remember that you are designing for both men and women, and that they might wish to do very different things outdoors.

- Consider providing several different outdoor areas if there are residents from very different backgrounds.

- Consider the faith needs of the residents, remembering that for many of the world religions, water has a special place and meaning.

- Beware of thinking in a limited way about outdoor space always as a garden—think of it as the 'room outside'.

Photo opposite: Volunteers and residents enjoy helping to care for the gardens at HammondCare, Miranda, Australia.

11
BUDGET, AFTERCARE AND ENGAGEMENT

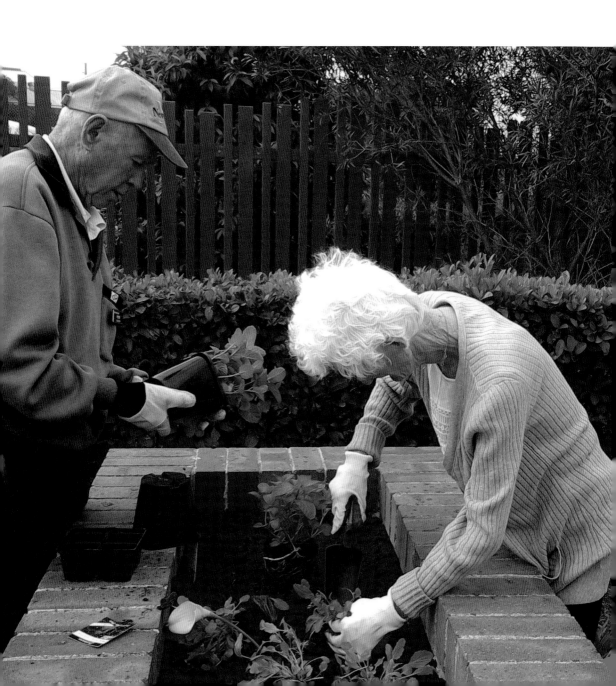

Protect outdoor budgets

Funding for your 'room outside' is often contained within the building budget. Sadly, examples of beautifully fitted-out buildings for people with dementia with no worthwhile garden are commonplace, because by the time outdoor spaces are considered, the budget has been used up.

As a result, outdoor spaces are often left as a sea of grass and boring, slabbed fire escape paths. This is a disaster!

Remember to think of the outdoor space as the 'room outside'—an essential part of the whole building environment. And try to secure and protect the landscape budget against building (and refurbishment) cost overruns.

Take a step back

The traditional approach for construction projects in the UK and most of Europe is where the client appoints a design team and tenders separately for a contractor when the design drawings are ready for pricing. This method allows for easy communication between the client and the design team and contractor as well as unbiased reports from the design team during the construction phase.

However, variations on a 'design-build' procurement route are increasingly being used in the UK and Europe, as well as Australian and New Zealand. This approach changes the traditional appointments and sequences of work. For the client, it provides a single point of responsibility in an attempt to reduce risks and overall costs (the same company both designs and builds the project). The main disadvantage of this

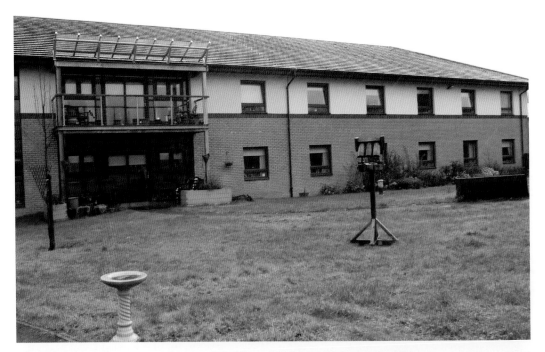

No budget for outdoors has resulted in a 'sea of grass' at this care home in the UK.
Photo: Richard Pollock

type of procurement is that the direct link between the design team and client no longer exists, which may result in an end product that has been affected by the contractor's primary concern to meet stringent cost considerations—and this may result in a less dementia inclusive end product.

Consequently, careful consideration of the type of procurement for the building and its outdoor spaces and ongoing communication between all parties is vital. Design for dementia must be foremost in considering what procurement route to follow.

Education matters

There are a number of options for the delivery of your landscape aftercare or maintenance, which include in-house staff and external contractors, or in some cases groups of volunteers who support your building e.g. the 'Friends of Crieff Hospital' or a local Rotary Group. Whichever option is chosen, it is important that the individuals responsible for maintenance are informed about the design intent of the outdoor spaces. Well-informed maintenance staff can help ensure that the design intent is maintained through the routine maintenance period, whereas individual interpretation of the landscape design may lead to unintended outcomes. For example, a maintenance team might allow a hedge to grow high, not realising that a low hedge was essential for visibility, to help minimise the risk of falls, confusion and injury.

A useful resource for informing maintenance staff is the development of a landscape design manual that explains the design intent in some detail. This important resource can be used during orientation of new staff, contractors and volunteers as well as ongoing support for existing staff and contractors.

Aftercare and maintenance costs

Routine or planned maintenance schedules are often forgotten or not prioritised during the transition from construction to operations. Good operational planning should always include a maintenance schedule with sufficient budget, detailing the frequency and cost of lawn mowing, pruning, weeding, mulching, fertilising, irrigation maintenance and plant replenishing. Not to be forgotten, is the regular cleaning and repairing of hard surfaces so that they are not hazardous.

Automated maintenance schedules are a good way of reminding when tasks are due and escalating when tasks are overdue. Failure to adhere to a comprehensive maintenance program costs money— normally far greater than if tasks are done on time. Like the design phase, a planned approach to maintenance activities actually saves money in the long run.[63]

When maintenance becomes engagement

As mentioned, maintenance and aftercare of outdoor spaces is usually the responsibility of a dedicated employee, group or an external contractor. Each context provides an important resource that can be used to support and engage with residents whose home it is. Many residents will have loved and cared for gardens or allotments in their life. While physical fitness may mean that more support is needed, this activity can be an important part of the person contributing to the life of their home, as well as an opportunity for fresh air and exercise!

Success in engaging and involving residents requires reconsideration of the staffing model and budget allocation. It may be beneficial to redirect budget set aside for 'activity or diversional therapy hours' into the maintenance budget. By supporting and training maintenance staff, it is possible to open a whole new area of meaningful engagement for people with dementia, as the following case study shows.

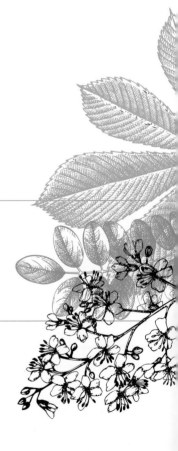

'Remember to think of the outdoor space as the "room outside"—an essential part of the whole building environment.'

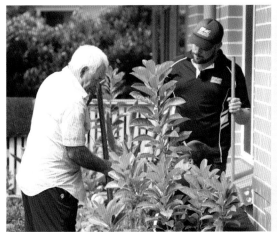
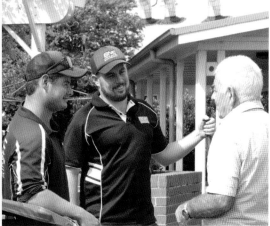

Involving Gus in garden maintenance, HammondCare, Hammondville, Australia.

Case study 9
Southwood Special Care Program—Hammondville, NSW, Australia.

Gus came to Australia from Italy as a young man and was a market gardener all his life. In his latter years dementia advanced quickly and with care options limited, he was placed in a psychogeriatric facility, much to the concern of family. Being outdoors was a key part of his life but 'outdoors' at this facility was a few square metres surrounded by high metal fences. It didn't feel like 'outdoors' to Gus. He was able to move into Linden Cottage where staff focused on getting to know Gus and how to best to enable him enjoy an improved quality of life. Easy access to outdoors and gardens is a key feature of Linden Cottage and this proved pivotal for supporting Gus.

The external garden maintenance team has been trained in communicating with and understanding the needs of people with dementia. Engaging with residents who want to participate in gardening or talk about the work is a key requirement of their contract, which ensures the task of garden maintenance is undertaken 'with' and not 'for' the person with dementia. This has resulted in a better outcome for everyone, in particular, Gus. He quickly took interest when the maintenance team came around and before long was equipped with a shovel to assist in planting, as well as hosing, raking and other gardening activities. The Special Care Program Manager acknowledged that there was some risk in giving a shovel to a strong and active man like Gus who had experienced distressed behaviours. 'But there's a risk in everything. There's a risk he could trip over on the concrete and fall. The bigger risk is to deny him the opportunity to help.'

Gus is clearly in his element, working alongside the contractors, with the gardening process a comforting and familiar pastime that promotes dignity and sense of identity.[64]

Key points

- Outdoor spaces, as with every other feature of buildings, are subject to wear and tear, as well as needing routine refreshing.

- Ensure the budget for maintaining the outdoor space has been secured. A garden lacking regular maintenance can look like a wasteland very quickly and this can deter people from using it.

- Linking the design, construction and maintenance processes can ensure the quality and intent of outdoor spaces is not lost over time.

- Involving maintenance staff in the initial design and explaining the reasons for particular plantings and design features can ensure there are no unintended consequences to maintenance activities. A landscape design manual may be helpful.

- Failing to have regular maintenance and aftercare will cost more in the long run.

12
MORE TIPS
FOR SUCCESS

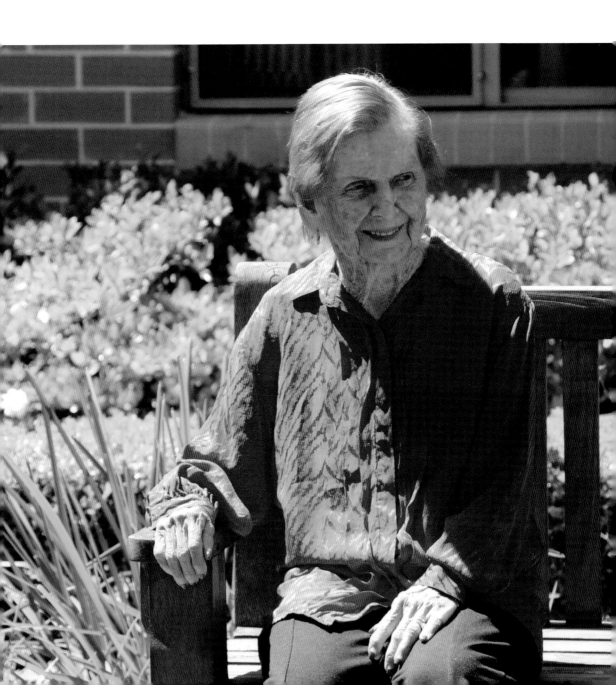

Developing a successful 'room outside' is a simple principle with often complex considerations. It's important to not just think of your outdoor spaces now, but to consider how they will grow and mature, and above all, how they relate to the human scale, i.e. not so large as to be intimidating, or so small as to feel cramped.

In addition to the wealth of advice and examples provided throughout *The room outside*, here's a further list of tips for helping you to achieve exceptional outdoor areas and gardens.

Design purposefully!

- Avoid a 'show garden' or 'signature' design—this kind of design is for looking at, not for using and working in.

- Think about how a person will relate to the scale of the outdoor space. If possible, it is worth getting 3D representations prepared, so that you can visualise and appreciate what you are getting at an early design stage—include sun access diagrams too.

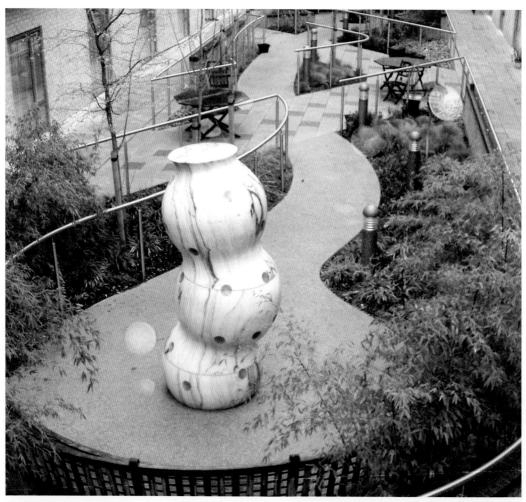

Don't design a show garden! Photo: Richard Pollock

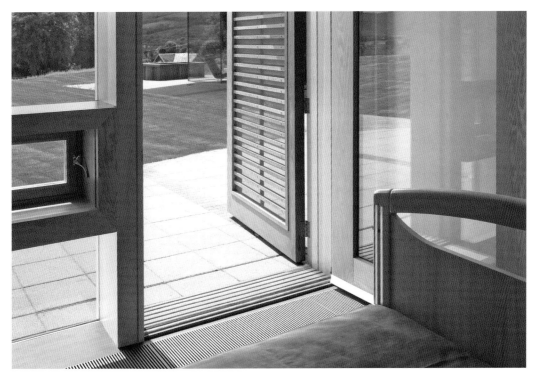

A door wide enough to allow a bed outside at Robin House Hospice, Balloch—Children's Hospice Association Scotland. Photo: Andrew Lee Photographer

Think about the views

As mentioned earlier, views can be absolutely vital to a person's mental wellbeing. An example of this was found in a geriatric ward in the new Enniskillen hospital in Northern Ireland. A patient, an elderly farmer with dementia, was showing distressed behaviour which often made providing care difficult for staff. Eventually they moved him to a room overlooking farmland. His behaviour and state of wellbeing improved dramatically.

Views can:
- encourage people outdoors

- provide valuable memory triggers of aspects of a person's early life and work

- help people recover from ill health faster.[65]

Soil is more than just dirt

- The structure of soil can be easily damaged by heavy machinery. Soil damage can lead to drainage issues resulting in plant deaths which are difficult to fix. Care must be taken during construction stage to minimise soil damage.

- Soil is acidic, neutral or alkaline (known as its pH value) and this can affect the type of plants that will thrive—it's worth testing so that you know what you have and can choose plants accordingly to suit the soil.

- Avoid spilling any pollutants on soil such as diesel—polluted soil may kill plants.

Welcoming wildlife and pets

Learn more about the wildlife in your area and consider pets too—both can provide lots of pleasure, but some creatures need to be managed or kept out:

- Birds, butterflies, small harmless lizards (in some countries) and even squirrels (although this will require 'squirrel-proof' bird feeders!) can provide much delight and encourage people to go outdoors. Possums, such as in Australia, might be interesting in a tree at night but they have a bad habit of getting into building roof spaces, causing unfortunate consequences!

- Some animals come in search of food, and may even be dangerous, for example, bears in North America.

- Pet rabbits are quite easy to care for and can be very tame, providing a great deal of enjoyment. However, wild rabbits can destroy a planting scheme in a short time, so if there are some around, rabbit-proof fencing is required to keep the planting safe.

- Cats, dogs, birds and farm animals can all give enormous pleasure, depending on the background and culture of your residents.

Think about your trees

Trees come in many sizes and forms, with varied types of foliage:

- Think about the ultimate size of trees and avoid planting them too close to buildings and windows. They can cause loss of light and possible structural damage within 10 to 20 years of planting and at that point, it can be expensive to remove the offending trees.

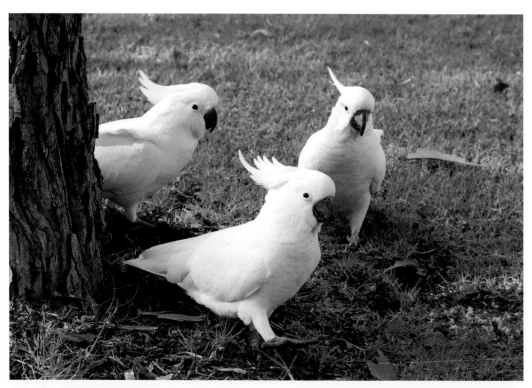

Friendly wildlife in Australia.

- Consider underground services when planting trees. Tree roots can cause damage, particularly to pipework, if there is not adequate protection.

- The need for shade varies according to climate—heavy shade may be really desirable in hot countries, yet highly undesirable in the northern latitudes.

- Look at the leaf, fruit and seed fall of trees: a heavy fall of leaves in the autumn can be slippery on the ground; fruits can stain paving, causing marks that can be disturbing to people with dementia; and heavy seeding trees are a maintenance burden when the many seed heads start to grow in the planting beds!

Caring for shrubs and plants

Plant descriptions can be very misleading—and many plants will need attention during the year:

- Dwarf shrubs are often not really dwarf size and end up needing 'haircuts' to keep them in shape, resulting in unattractive blocks of planting. Do the research and also ensure that they are pruned and shaped appropriately and not just dealt with by a chainsaw!

- Herbaceous plants can be interesting and variable, but often need splitting and repositioning after a few years. This can be a bonus as you get plants for 'free'— but if not done, the appearance can suffer.

- Some plants are really very aggressive and best avoided—seek expert advice.

- Every plant needs fertilising annually to keep healthy, don't skimp on maintenance.

Final word—enjoy the adventure together

Designing outdoor spaces for older people and people with dementia is not only rewarding, but an adventure to be shared. A key aspect is 'knowing' the people you are seeking to support through your design, hearing their voice and understanding their needs. Learning more about your resident groups, clients or patients is vital and enjoyable and will involve listening to their comments, advice and stories as well as those of their families and friends. This will help to ensure appropriate design that works well and improves quality of life.

Another key aspect is involving the staff/carers in plans for the outdoor spaces. When they understand the importance of the 'room outside' it is more likely they will help the people they are caring for to access the outdoors freely and partake in outdoor activities.

Also, of particular importance is receiving ongoing feedback and sharing with others your knowledge of what has worked well and what hasn't. In this way, designing outdoor spaces for people with dementia can only get better.

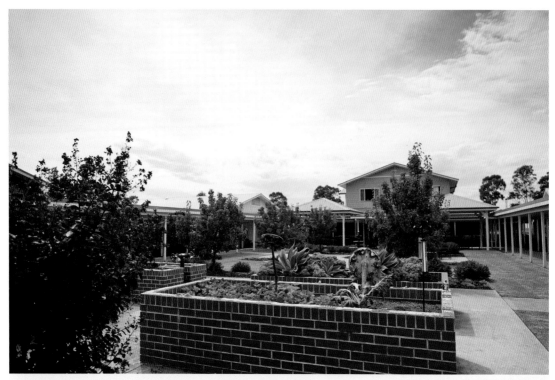

Raised garden beds, HammondCare, Horsley, Australia.

Case study 10
Hierarchical spacing—Horsley, Australia.

HammondCare Horsley is an aged care home consisting of six single storey cottages, each home to 15 residents—many who have a diagnosis of dementia. The cottages are arranged around a courtyard which links them all and provides a useful shared outside space.

Horsley's site layout is a good example of a hierarchical arrangement of external spaces which progress naturally from the main entrance area (publicly accessible), through the common courtyard (shared by all residents), then to each front garden (accessible to all residents, but 'belonging' to individual cottages), and, finally, the private backyard (accessible to just those 15 residents and their guests).

The main courtyard space is designed like a formal park, a design residents find to be recognisable and familiar. While completely enclosed and secure, there is no feeling of being 'contained' due to the scale of the courtyard, and the lack of visible boundary.

Its design makes it obvious that it is for communal use, and its regular layout makes it easy to navigate. It has hedging and ordered pathways and a decorative, traditional fountain at the centre is a major orientating landmark. This spot is popular with residents who often sit close by and watch the numerous birds that come to bathe in the water.

From this courtyard, residents can freely access several amenities:

- A well-equipped barbecue area is used weekly for group events run by staff, residents and volunteers. Families can use this area on the weekend, and there is good shading to make it useable in a variety of weathers.

- One area has raised garden beds—used by volunteers and residents for vegetable gardening. Beside this area is a well-equipped maintenance shed where residents and families can access tools for gardening and odd-jobs around the grounds. People are encouraged to get involved as much as they want.

- The planting is mainly deciduous, and there is good seasonal change, helpful for orientating residents who may be less sure of the passage of time. A highlight of the year is September when the beautiful apple blossom comes into full bloom.

The cottage back gardens cottages are tailored to the preferences of the residents who live there. An example is a cottage garden where one of the gazebos was converted to an art studio. One of the residents is an avid artist and enjoys painting there in the garden almost every day.[66]

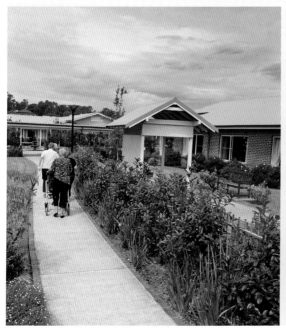
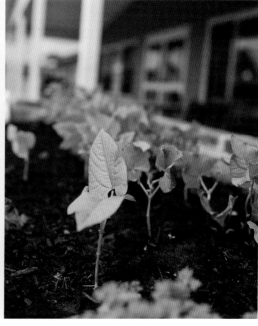

APPENDIX—
PERSONAL EXPERIENCES

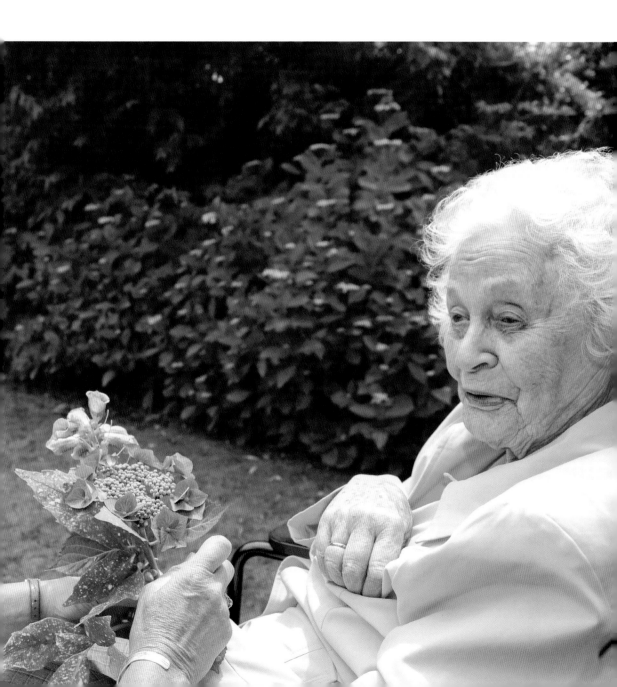

Appendix—Personal experiences

In *The room outside* we have discussed the extensive range of needs that can be met and the benefits received when outdoor spaces are incorporated in the care of older people and people with dementia. And we have sought to enable implementation of this knowledge through providing practical tips and design recommendations. The stories you are about to read show you the frontline effect of the outdoor space on both the carer and the person with dementia. The importance of 'rooms outside' cannot be underestimated, nor can the positive impact they have on the person with dementia.

***

Catherine* is a sprightly 93-year-old who comes out with me in the car twice a week. She is living with Alzheimer's, has a very poor short-term memory, is a little hard of hearing and sometimes has difficulty finding the right words. Her eyesight, however, is very good and she has a wicked sense of humour. She prefers peace and quiet so we usually drive down to the sea front, sit in the car, look at all that's going on and have a conversation. When she first gets in the car she often says how lovely it is sitting in the front seat and being able to see everything. While I'm driving she will comment on the planes going over, the amount of cars she sees on the road, the size of the trucks and lorries, how many red or green lights there are at junctions, in fact she misses little of what we pass by.

When we arrive at the sea front and park, Catherine will comment on how peaceful it is. She points out the jet streams of airplanes, the different colours of the water and observes whether the water is calm or choppy. She remarks on the formation of the clouds, especially if there are dark ones moving towards us, and bright lights or other objects she notices on the far horizon. I often use my binoculars so Catherine will ask me to identify something she can see but doesn't recognise. She will count the number of carriages of the trains going over the rail bridge, and will notice the different types of vehicles going over the road bridge, especially the weird shape of the car transporters.

Sometimes I will notice a particular kind of bird through my binoculars, look it up in my book and show her what it is and where I've seen it. We will often read some of the description of the birds together.

Sometimes, weather permitting, we will have a walk along the promenade. On one occasion we were standing at the railing (Catherine loves the colour of blue they are painted) looking out over the water, with the sun behind us. Suddenly she said 'there we are' and pointed down towards the little patch of muddy ground below. She had noticed our reflections in the puddles and so I waved, she did the same and both of us giggled at the absurdity of waving at ourselves. This is how much joy being outdoors brought us both.
From Margaret, carer, Scotland

***

Mary and Joan* are two residents of a dementia cottage who share a similar background and enjoy spending time together. One day Mary's family visited and because there were two small children, it was decided to head into the garden to enjoy the autumn sun.

Mary invited Joan to join them and after a walk along the path, including a rest at the gazebo, the whole group sat on the outdoor furniture near the entrance to the 'outside room' and watched the children playing. A claret ash was displaying beautiful colour and the children, laughing, began throwing the fallen leaves in the air and before long were playfully scattering them over Mary and Joan, to everyone's delight. A volunteer brought a therapy dog to visit and this added to the excitement—all bathed in beautiful warm sun.

There was no stress about what the children might get up to as the outdoor space was large enough for expending lots of energy, has excellent sight lines, level paths and was subtly enclosed. When it was time for family to go, both Mary and Joan, thoughtfully, had a turn at sweeping up the leaves left behind and then adjourned inside for a cup of tea.

While family are welcome to visit any time and there are various indoor spaces available, access to the outdoors added rich levels of engagement, reminiscence and even seasonal prompts, all the while gaining some healthy vitamin D!
From Andrew, volunteer, Australia

***

Valerie* is a physically active woman in her late seventies who is living with Alzheimer's. She has a poor short-term memory and difficulty finding the right words, but has good hearing and eyesight and loves to go out. Her favourite places include along the river in Cramond, the Water of Leith, the Botanic Garden, Craigie Farm and garden centres. She loves meeting people and their dogs, and watching children at play. She quite spontaneous when it comes to starting conversations with complete strangers.

Valerie notices and comments on the construction of old stone walls and buildings as often as the trees and shrubs we pass. She will notice the detail of leaves on trees and shrubs and will often ask me if I know what they are, expecting me to know and gently chastising me if I don't. I also have books on trees and wild flowers in the car as well as a mobile phone with internet so I can usually find the answer and then Valerie enthusiastically compliments me on my vast knowledge.

I am often surprised by Valerie's attention to the detailed patterns of leaves on trees, their trunks, their overall shape and height. She notices and comments on bird song and will stand and patiently watch birds flying around in the woods, or will use the feeders in a garden centre. Recently Valerie was enchanted by a young bird flying closely around us and finally settling on her outstretched hand. Her smile said it all.

Valerie loves to sing and often bursts into a particular song when we link arms to start a walk. We have brought smiles to a few faces while out walking and we also sing in the car, particularly on our return home.

Not only does the outdoor space enable her to have a quality of life that doesn't rely on the impairments caused by dementia, but it also provides her with a moment of connection—free from distress and confusion.

From Margaret, carer, Scotland

***

Gerard* is one of several residents who enjoy engaging in a community 'Friendship Garden' established at his Melbourne (Australia) nursing home. A local gardening group established the age-appropriate gardens with support from nursing home management and visit regularly each month to care for the gardens with help from residents with a love of gardening. As well, local school students are invited to visit and engage with residents and the garden in activities carefully planned to be meaningful and enjoyable for all involved. Drawing alongside a raised garden bed in his wheelchair, Gerard can be seen chatting with the students and giving them advice as they undertake gardening activities. So successful is interaction in the Friendship Garden that it featured in a photo exhibition of significant local gardens. This showcased the value of gardens and outdoors spaces in providing not only a healthy and enjoyable activity for aged care residents, but in being an intergenerational point of connection with the local community.

From Kylie, manager, Victoria.

Tell us your stories

We'd love to hear your stories about the personal impact of outdoors spaces and the unique ways they play a role in the care and support of older people and people living with dementia. Email us at theroomoutside@hammond.com.au and we'll include the best stories on our room outside web forum.

*Names changed to protect privacy.

REFERENCES

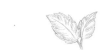

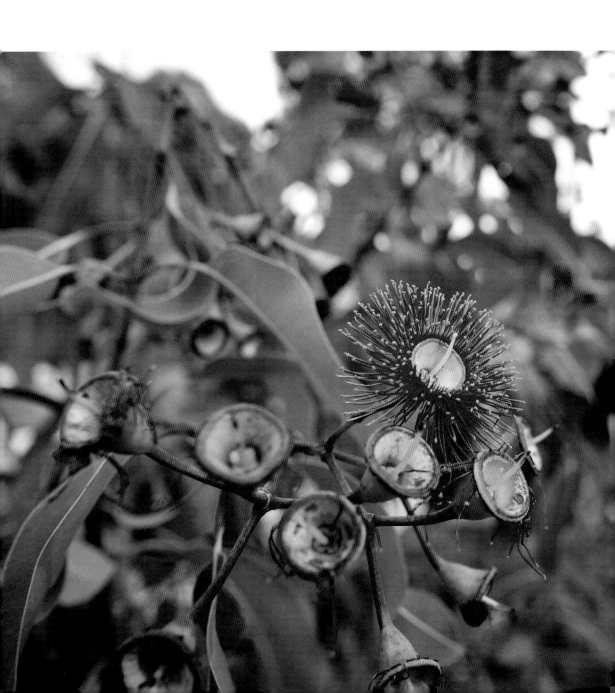

Introduction

[1]R Potter, B Sheehan, R Cain, J Griffin & P A Jennings, 'The Impact of the Physical Environment on Depressive Symptoms of Older Residents Living in Care Homes: A Mixed Methods Study', *Gerontologist*, gnx041, 2017, viewed 25 July 2017, <https://academic.oup.com/gerontologist/article/doi/10.1093/geront/gnx041/3848859/The-Impact-of-the-Physical-Environment-on>.

01 Impairments of dementia and older age

[2]Dementia and Sensory Challenges, ed. A Houston, 2016.

[3]S Macfarlane & C Cunningham, 'The need for holistic management of behavioral disturbances in dementia', International *Psychogeriatrics*, vol. 29, no. 7, 2017, pp. 1055-1058.

[4]Macfarlane & Cunningham, pp.1055-1058

[5]*Dementia and Sensory Challenges*, ed. A Houston, 2016.

[6]*About us*, Dementia Support Australia, AU, 2017, viewed June 8 2017, <http://dementia.com.au/about/>.

02 Going outside is good for us

[7]L Teri, RG Logsdon & SM McCurry, 'Exercise Interventions for Dementia and Cognitive Impairment: The Seattle Protocols', *The Journal of Nutrition, Health & Aging*, vol. 2, no. 6, 2008, pp. 391-394.

[8]H Godman, *Regular exercise changes the brain to improve memory*, Harvard Health Publications, Boston, Massachusetts, 2014, updated 2016, viewed February 18 2017, <http://www.health.harvard.edu/blog/regular-exercise-changes-brain-improve-memory-thinking-skills-201404097110>.

[9]T Fukushima, K Nagahata, N Ishibashi, Y Takahashi & M Moriyama, 'Quality of life from the viewpoint of patients with dementia in Japan: nurturing through an acceptance of dementia by patients, their families and care professionals', *Health & Social Care in the Community*, vol. 13, no. 1, 2005, pp. 30-7.

[10]S Duggan, T Blackman, A Martyr, PV Schaik, 'The impact of early dementia on outdoor life: A "shrinking world"?', *Dementia*, vol. 7, no. 2, 2008, pp.191-204.

[11]F Wright & RB Weller, 'Risks and benefits of UV radiation in older people: More of a friend than a foe?,' *Maturitas*, vol. 81, no. 4, 2015, pp. 425-31.

[12]Wright and Weller, p. 425.

[13]*UVA and UVB*, The Skin Cancer Foundation, NY, 2016, viewed February 6 2017, <http://www.skincancer.org/prevention/uva-and-uvb>.

[14]Multiple Sclerosis-UK Limited, *MS-UK*, Colchester, Essex, 2016, viewed February 6 2017, <http://www.ms-uk.org/files/choices_vitd.pdf>.

[15]D McNair, R Pollock & C Cunningham, *Enlighten*, HammondCare Media, Sydney, November 2017.

[16]*Vitamin D Council*, San Luis Obispo, CA, 2016, viewed February 6 2017, <http://www.vitamindcouncil.org>.

[17]*Vitamin D*, Cancer Council Australia, Sydney, NSW, 2016, viewed June 5 2017, <http://www.cancer.org.au/preventing-cancer/sun-protection/vitamin-d>.

[18]F Wright & RB Weller, 'Risks and benefits of UV radiation in older people: More of a friend than a foe?', *Maturitas*, vol. 81, no. 4, 2015, pp. 425-31.

[19]Richard Weller, 'Could the sun be good for your heart?', TED - Ideas worth spreading, 2012, viewed February 5 2017, <https://www.ted.com/talks/richard_weller_could_the_sun_be_good_for_your_heart?language=en#>.

[20]ST Kent, LA McClure, WL Crosson, DK Arnett, VG Wadley & N Sathiakumar, 'Effect of sunlight exposure on cognitive function among depressed and non-depressed participants: a REGARDS cross-sectional study', *Environmental Health*, vol. 8, no. 34, 2009, viewed July 25 2017, <http://dx.doi.org/10.1186/1476-069X-8-34>.

[21]Mind, Ecotherapy, *The green agenda for mental health*, Mind publications, UK, 2013, viewed July 1 2017, <https://www.mind.org.uk/media/273470/ecotherapy.pdf>.

[22]Natural England Commissioned Report NECR211, *Is it nice outside? - Consulting people living with dementia and their carers about engaging with the natural environment*, Natural England, UK, 2016.

[23]CJ Wood, J Pretty & M Griffin, 'A case-control study of the health and well-being benefits of allotment gardening', *Journal of Public Health*, vol. 38, no. 3, 2015, viewed June 8 2017, <https://academic.oup.com/jpubhealth/article-abstract/38/3/e336/2239844/A-case-control-study-of-the-health-and-well-being>.

[24]Drug and Therapeutics Bulletin Editorial Office, 'Management of seasonal affective disorder,' *BMJ*, vol. 340, 2010.

[25]RN Golden, BN Gaynes, RD Ekstrom, RM Hamer, FM Jacobsen, T Suppes, KL Wisner & CB Nemeroff, 'The efficacy of light therapy in the treatment of mood disorders: A review and meta-analysis of the evidence', *The American journal of psychiatry*, vol. 162, no. 4, 2005, pp. 656-62.

[26]E Urrestarazu & J Iriarte, 'Clinical management of sleep disturbances in Alzheimer's disease: current and emerging strategies', *Nature and Science of Sleep*, vol. 8, 2016, viewed February 6 2017, <doi: 10.2147/NSS.S76706>.

[27]EB Larson, L Wang, JD Bowen, WV McCormick, L Teri, L Crane P & W Kukull, 'Exercise is associated with reduced risk for incident dementia among persons 65 years of age and older', *American College of Physicians*, vol. 144, no. 2, 2006, pp. 73-81.

[28]T Burrell, 'Circuit train your brain', *New Scientist*, vol. 227, no. 3035, 2015, pp. 32-37.

[29]JL Etnier, PM Nowell, DM Landers & BA Sibley, 'A meta-regression to examine the relationship between aerobic fitness and cognitive performance', *Brain research reviews*, vol. 52, no. 1, 2006, pp. 119-30.

[30]C Marlene, 'Rising Outdoor CO2 Levels Harming Life Indoors (Op-Ed)', LiveScience, New York, 2016, viewed April 25 2016, <http://www.livescience.com/52619-indoor-air-quality-affects-how-your-mind-functions.html>.

[31]*Dignity and respect: dementia continuing care visits*, Mental Welfare Commission for Scotland, Edinburgh, 2014.

[32]TL Scott, *Examining the therapeutic effect of gardens and gardening activities for older adults residing in the community and in aged-care facilities*, University of Qld, Qld, 2012, viewed June 8 2017, <https://espace.library.uq.edu.au/view/UQ:302191>.

[33]D Carroll & M Rendell, *The Care Culture Map and Handbook*, Step Change Design Ltd, Southampton, 2016, viewed April 16 2017, <http://www.stepchange-design.co.uk/wp-content/uploads/2016/07/NAPA-Living-Life-Autumn14.pdf>.

[34]Information supplied by Diane Gardiner, Interim Head of Nursing POA (in-patients) and Senior Charge Nurse Ward One, Dementia Assessment Unit, Crieff Community Hospital, Scotland.

03 Planning for 'rooms outside'

[35]*Greenweb*, Sutherland Shire Council, NSW, 2015 viewed June 8 2017, <http://www.sutherlandshire.nsw.gov.au/Outdoors/Environment/Plants-and-Bushland/Greenweb>.

[36]*Environmental benefits of greenspace – Noise abatement*, Forestry Research, UK, 2017, viewed June 1 2017, <https://www.forestry.gov.uk/fr/infd-8aefl5>.

[37]G Plascencia-Villa, A Ponce, JF Collingwood, MJ Arellano-Jimenez, X Zhu, JT Rogers, I Betancourt, M Jose-Yacaman & G Perry, 'High-resolution analytical imaging and electron holography of magnetite particles in amyloid cores of Alzheimer's disease', Scientific Reports, vol. 6, no. 24873, 2016, viewed February 6, 2017, <https://www.ncbi.nlm.nih.gov/pmc/articles/PMC4848473/>.

[38]CR Jung, YT Lin & BF Hwang, 'Ozone, particulate matter, and newly diagnosed Alzheimer's disease: a population-based cohort study in Taiwan', *Journal of Alzheimer's disease*, vol. 44, no. 2, 2015, pp. 573-84.

[39]RG Donovan, HE Stewart, SM Owen, AP Mackenzie & N Hewitt, 'Development and Application of an Urban Tree Air Quality Score for Photochemical Pollution Episodes Using the Birmingham, United Kingdom, Area as a Case Study', *Environmental Science & Technology*, vol. 39, 2005, viewed February 5 2017, <http://www.es.lancs.ac.uk/people/cnh/UrbanTreesBrochure.pdf>.

[40]KV Abhijith, P Kumar, J Gallagher, Aonghus McNabola, R Baldauf, F Pilla, B Broderick, S Di Sababino & B Pulvirentia, 'Air pollution abatement performances of green infrastructure in open road and built up street canyon environments – a review', *Atmospheric Environment*, vol. 162, 2017, viewed June 25 2017, <https://doi.org/10.1016/j.atmosenv.2017.05.014>.

[41]P Whatt, '99-year-old says controversial care home Oakland in Swadlincote is "out of this world"', *Derby Telegraph*, UK, 2013, viewed January 25 2017, <http://www.derbytelegraph.co.uk/99-year-old-says-controversial-care-home-Oakland/story-18469316-detail/story.html#ixzz41BTMs02n>.

04 Developing a range of activities

[42]*Is it nice outside? - Consulting people living with dementia and their carers about engaging with the natural environment* (NECR211), Natural England, UK, 2016, viewed February 6 2017, <http://publications.naturalengland.org.uk/publication/5910641209507840>.

[43]G Chalfont & A Walker, Dementia Green Care Handbook of Therapeutic Design and Practice, Safehouse Books, Arizona, 2013.

[44]DSDC, *The Creating Conversations Kit: Gardening*, University of Stirling, UK, 2012, viewed April 21, 2017, <http://www.creating-conversations.org>.

[45]Information supplied by 3 Bridges Care Home Director, Margaret Sawyer.

[46]Information supplied by family visitor, Peter.

05 Design that helps people get outside

[47]E Rappe & SL Kivela, 'Effects of Garden Visits on Long-term Care Residents as Related to Depression', *Hort Technology*, vol. 15, 2005, pp.194-195.

06 Safe and inviting 'rooms outside'

[48]M Marshall, Designing balconies, roof terraces and roof gardens for people with dementia, Dementia Services Development Centre, University of Stirling, United Kingdom, 2010.

[49]RS Ulrich, 'View through a window may influence recovery from surgery', *Science*, vol. 224, no. 4647, 1984, viewed February 6 2017, <https://mdc.mo.gov/sites/default/files/resources/2012/10/ulrich.pdf>.

07 Furniture and structures

[50]As described by a residential care manger at Strathearn House, Scone, NSW, Australia.

[51]Information supplied by Solardome® Industries.

10 Cultural and spiritual considerations

[52]*Designing outdoor spaces for people with dementia*, ed. Annie Pollock and Mary Marshall, HammondCare Media and Dementia Services Development Centre, the University of Stirling, 2012.

[53]World Urbanisation Prospects (Highlights)—United Nations, viewed June 1, 2017, https://esa.un.org/unpd/wup/Publications/Files/WUP2014-Highlights.pdf

[54]John 15:1, New Testament, Holy Bible.

[55]G Otte, 'The Ismaili Centre opens its doors to Londoners', *The Ismaili*, 2017, viewed February 13 2017, <http://www.theismaili.org/news-events/opens-its-doors-londoners>.

[56]H Wieringa & S Attia, '"Islamic garden in Christian world", "Christian garden in Islamic world"—A research paper about cross cultural perspective in the age of global architectural practice', Wageningen University, Department of Environmental Design, School of Landscape, Architecture, *Design Theory Spring*, 2005, viewed June 7 2017.

[57]'Native American' from the *Federal Bureau of Prisoners' Technical Reference Manual on Innate Beliefs and Practices*, 2002, http://ccky.org/wp-content/uploads/2011/06/Native-American. pdf, viewed January 26, 2017.

[58]J Korff, *Aboriginal spirituality and beliefs*, Creative Spirits, Australia, 2016, viewed March 5 2016, <http://www.creativespirits.info/aboriginalculture/spirituality/#axzz421YUtXiD>.

[59]*Take 2: Housing Design in Indigenous Australia*, ed. Paul Memmott, The Royal Australian Institute of Architects, Red Hill, ACT, 2003.

[60]DW Hamacher & RP Norris, *'Bridging the Gap' through Australian Cultural Astronomy*, Cambridge University Press, Cambridge, England, 2011.

[61]Ray & Cilla Norris, *Emu dreaming: An Introduction to Australian Aboriginal Astronomy*, Emu Dreaming, Australia, 2009.

[62]Information supplied by Liz Fuggle. Planning Officer, Architect, HammondCare

11 Budget, aftercare and engagement

[63]Maintenance information supplemented by Michael Cooney, General Manager, Property and Capital Works, HammondCare.

[64]Information supplied by Colm Cunningham and also the 'Gus Spezza's Story' video, viewed June 30, 2017, <https://youtu.be/JPSMa8yqT7o>.

12 More tips for success

[65]RS Ulrich, 'View through a window may influence recovery from surgery', *Science*, New/series, vol. 224, issue 4647, 1984, pp. 420-421.

[66]Information supplied by Liz Fuggle, Planning Officer, Architect, HammondCare

Further reading

CC Marcus and N Sachs, *Therapeutic Landscapes, An Evidence-Based Approach to Designing Healing Gardens and Restorative Outdoor Spaces*, Wiley, Hoboken, New Jersey, 2014.

Culturally Appropriate Outside Spaces and Experiences for People with Dementia, ed. Mary Marshall and Jane Gilliard, Jessica Kingsley, London, UK, 2014.

Designing outdoor spaces for people with dementia, ed. Annie Pollock and Mary Marshall, HammondCare Media and Dementia Services Development Centre, the University of Stirling, 2012.

Grefsrod and A Eek, *Gardens for people with dementia*, Aldring og helse [Ageing and Health], Norway, 2008.

Outdoor Environments for People with Dementia, ed. Susan Rodiek and Benjamin Schwarz, Taylor and Francis Inc, New York, 2008.

TG Cochrane, *Gardens that Care: Planning Outdoor Environments for People with Dementia*, Alzheimer's Australia, South Australia, AU, 2010.

G Chalfont, *Dementia Green Care, Design Guide*, Chalfont Design, Sheffield, UK, 2012.

Transforming the Quality of Life for People with Dementia through Contact with the Natural World, ed. Jane Gilliard and Mary Marshall, Jessica Kingsley, London, UK, 2012.

Acknowledgements

Enormous thanks to all the following people who have helped and been very supportive in the writing of this book:

- Emeritus Professor Mary Marshall, Senior Consultant, HammondCare, for reviewing and providing guidance throughout

- Liz Fuggle, Planning Officer and Architect, HammondCare, for commenting and editing

- Ricky Pollock, Associate Consultant, Architect, HammondCare, for his support in proof reading, providing photographs and looking at references

- David McNair, Associate Consultant, Light and Lighting, HammondCare, for his contribution on lighting and providing references

- Richard Weller, Associate Principal Investigator, Centre for Inflammation Research, University of Edinburgh, for his help on vitamin D and nitric oxide

- Iain Stewart, Edinburgh Inter-Faith Association, for providing help in finding out about faith and garden areas and all those who responded through him

- Michael Cooney, General Manager of Property and Capital Works, HammondCare, for insights into outdoor maintenance and aftercare

- Mrs Kulwinder S Kusbia of the Edinburgh Sikh community

- Nila Joshi of the Edinburgh Hindu community

- Iqbal Hussein, Part 2 graduate in architecture, for advice on Islam

- Umi Osakabe, Architect, BPA-Architecture, for advice on Japanese garden design.

- Margaret Robertson, carer in Edinburgh

- The HammondCare Media team for editing and publishing services.

About the authors

Annie Pollock (Architect and Landscape Architect) is an Associate Consultant for HammondCare and previously provided consultancy services for the Dementia Services Development Centre at Stirling University.

As an architect, she worked on housing, hospital and airport design, before undertaking further studies in Landscape Architecture, a career that she has followed since.

In her Edinburgh-based Landscape Architecture practice 'Arterre', Annie has specialised for more than 40 years in designing outdoor spaces for older people. She has won several awards for her work, including a Royal Horticultural Show Silver Medal for the 'Forget me not Garden' for Alzheimer Scotland and Action on Dementia, Strathclyde Country Park (1999); a British Association of Landscape Industries (BALI) award, jointly with the contractor, for the courtyard garden at the Iris Murdoch Building, University of Stirling (2003) and a British Urban Regeneration Association (BURA) commended award for Dumbiedykes Estate regeneration, Edinburgh (2008).

Annie is passionate about design for older people and those with dementia—and has spoken internationally on both building and outdoor space design. She has also provided consultancy and training services extensively throughout the UK and in Europe, China and Australia.

Annie is widely published and publications include *Designing Gardens for People with Dementia, Air Quality and Health for People with Dementia and the Design for People with Dementia Audit Tool* (published by the University of Stirling in 2001, 2008 and 2015 respectively), Contributions to Lost in Space, 2014 and Not another Care handbook 2014 for the *Journal of Dementia Care*. She also edited and contributed to Designing Outdoor Spaces for People with Dementia, published in 2012, jointly by the University of Stirling and HammondCare.

She was recently part of a team providing guidance for HammondCare's 'Design online', an internet-based tool which advises both staff and designers on the best dementia-enabling design for inside and outdoor spaces.

Colm Cunningham, Director of the Dementia Centre, HammondCare, Colm leads an Australian and International team of over 200 staff involved in research, education and consultancy as well as the translation of this knowledge into accessible publications and tools to improve practice. The centre's priorities are building design, life engagement, models of care, understanding behaviour and end of life care. Colm is an international expert with over 30 years' experience in older age care. Colm leads national dementia behaviour response services, Dementia Support Australia, with the aim of reconsidering what it means to have a 'behaviour of concern'. A general and intellectual disability nurse and social worker, Colm was the deputy director at the UK Dementia Centre, University of Stirling and has written extensively and undertaken research on a wide range of issues about dementia including design, pain care, hospital care, night time care and intellectual disability. Working across a range of faculties of education and research in HammondCare, Colm has significant expertise in supporting translational research and meaningful practice and culture change. Colm is a Conjoint Associate Professor at the University of New South Wales School of Public Health and Community Medicine and a Visiting Fellow in Dementia Design and Practice at the University of Edinburgh School of Health in Social Science. Colm is also a member of the Wicking Strategic Review Panel.

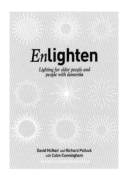

Enlighten

Light and lighting that promotes health and independence doesn't just happen. It needs to be designed, with awareness of the specific needs of older people and people with dementia. *Enlighten* provides both general insights for a broad readership and detailed technical information for engineers, architects and designers responsible for new buildings, refurbishments and alterations.

Enlighten explains how much light is enough, why access to natural light benefits health and how contrast, colour and reflection can hinder or support us in making sense of our world.

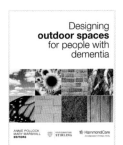

Designing outdoor spaces for people with dementia

Designing Outdoor Spaces for People with Dementia is edited by internationally respected experts Mary Marshall and Annie Pollock. Featuring authors from Japan, USA, Norway, the UK as well as Australia, the book provides a review of evidence-based research supporting the importance of access to outdoor spaces, tips on understanding how to use outdoor spaces appropriately and case studies from around the world describing how to develop and utilise well designed spaces for people with dementia.

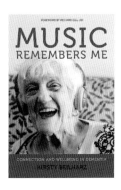

Music remembers me

Music remembers me: Connection and wellbeing in dementia brings to life the experience of people living with dementia and their interaction with music through an Australian-first project involving more than 700 aged care residents. While a diagnosis of dementia may be stressful and challenging, this book equips people living with dementia and those who support them with positive, meaningful ways of using music to enjoy experiences together-maximising feeling and connection.